HIV PREVENTION AND AWARENESS:

A VITAL HANDBOOK

DR. MELISSA P. NELSON

TABLE OF CONTENTS

PREFACE

In a world filled with information, there are topics that demand our attention and our action. HIV/AIDS is undeniably one of them.

Welcome to "HIV Prevention and Awareness: A Vital Handbook." Within these pages, we embark on a journey together—a journey to understand, prevent, and combat one of the most significant health challenges of our time.

HIV/AIDS is more than just a virus; it's a story of resilience, advocacy, and compassion. It's a global issue that transcends borders, affecting millions of lives regardless of age, gender, race, or sexual orientation. It's a call to action, a reminder that knowledge is power and that by arming ourselves with information, we can create a safer, more compassionate world.

This handbook is a compass, guiding you through the intricate terrain of HIV prevention and awareness. Whether you are seeking to safeguard your own health, support a loved one, or become an advocate for change, these pages hold the tools and insights you need.

We delve into the science, history, and impact of HIV/AIDS, exploring the latest developments in prevention and treatment. We address the stigmas and challenges that persist, urging you to join us in dismantling them. We share stories of strength and resilience, reminding you that hope and positivity are integral to the fight against HIV/AIDS.

Through knowledge, empathy, and collaboration, we can turn the tide against HIV/AIDS. This handbook is your companion in that endeavor, equipping you with the knowledge and resources to make a difference. It is a testament to the power of awareness, compassion, and collective action.

So, as you turn the pages of "HIV Prevention and Awareness: A Vital Handbook," remember that you are not alone in this journey. Together, we can raise awareness, prevent transmission, and support those affected by HIV/AIDS. Together, we can build a healthier, more inclusive world.

Thank you for taking the first step. Welcome to a world of knowledge, compassion, and hope.

CHAPTER 1: INTRODUCTION TO HIV/AIDS

Human Immunodeficiency Virus (HIV) and Acquired Immunodeficiency Syndrome (AIDS) are two closely related yet distinct conditions that have had a profound impact on public health, society, and individuals around the world. HIV is a virus that attacks the immune system, while AIDS is the advanced stage of HIV infection when the immune system is severely damaged. In this introduction, we will provide a brief overview of the history of the HIV/AIDS epidemic, its global prevalence and impact, and the importance of HIV prevention and awareness.

A Brief History of the HIV/AIDS Epidemic

The HIV/AIDS epidemic is one of the most devastating public health crises of the 20th and 21st centuries. Its history is marked by a complex interplay of scientific discovery, social stigma, and global response efforts. Here's a condensed overview of the key milestones in the history of the HIV/AIDS epidemic:

Early Cases and Identification (1980s):

The first recognized cases of AIDS (Acquired Immunodeficiency Syndrome) appeared in the early 1980s, primarily among gay men in the United States. Doctors noticed a cluster of rare diseases and infections in previously healthy individuals.

In 1983, two research teams independently identified the virus responsible for AIDS: the Human Immunodeficiency Virus (HIV). This discovery paved the way for understanding the disease's transmission and progression.

Rapid Spread and Stigmatization (1980s):

The virus quickly spread beyond the initial affected populations, including intravenous drug users, hemophiliacs, and heterosexual individuals.

HIV/AIDS was initially stigmatized, leading to discrimination and misconceptions about its transmission, contributing to the social isolation of affected individuals.

Global Impact (1980s–1990s):

The 1980s and 1990s saw the epidemic's rapid global expansion. SubSaharan Africa, in particular, was severely affected, with millions of people becoming infected and dying.

The lack of access to treatment, healthcare infrastructure, and education exacerbated the crisis in many parts of the world.

Scientific Advances (1990s):

In the mid-1990s, the development of antiretroviral therapy (ART) revolutionized HIV/AIDS treatment. ART could suppress the virus, slow disease progression, and prolong life.

Research into HIV transmission, prevention methods (e.g., condom use, needle exchange programs), and the development of preexposure prophylaxis (PrEP) further advanced our understanding of the virus.

Global Response (2000–Present):

International organizations, governments, and NGOs have initiated comprehensive efforts to combat HIV/AIDS. The United Nations established UNAIDS to coordinate global responses.

The 2000s and 2010s saw significant progress in expanding access to HIV testing, treatment, and prevention programs, particularly in high-prevalence regions.

Awareness campaigns aimed at reducing stigma and discrimination against people living with HIV/AIDS gained momentum.

Ongoing Challenges and Hope (Present):

HIV/AIDS remains a global challenge, with millions of people living with the virus. However, advances in treatment, prevention, and research offer hope for controlling the epidemic.

Key challenges include reaching vulnerable and marginalized populations, addressing disparities in access to healthcare, and continuing efforts to reduce stigma.

Research into potential HIV cures and vaccines continues, offering the possibility of ending the epidemic once and for all.

In summary, the history of the HIV/AIDS epidemic is a story of both tragedy and resilience. While it has caused immense suffering and loss, it has also spurred scientific innovation, advocacy, and global collaboration. The fight against HIV/AIDS is ongoing, with a commitment to prevention, treatment, and awareness as essential components of the effort to control and ultimately eradicate the virus.

Global Prevalence and Impact of HIV/AIDS

HIV/AIDS is a global pandemic that has had a profound and far-reaching impact on individuals, communities, and nations around the world. As of my last knowledge update in September 2021, here is an overview of the global prevalence and impact of HIV/AIDS:

- **Prevalence:**

Global HIV Infections: An estimated 38 million people worldwide were living with HIV in 2020.

New Infections: There were approximately 1.5 million new HIV infections in 2020.

AIDS-Related Deaths: In the same year, around 680,000 people died from AIDS-related illnesses.

- **Regional Disparities:**

SubSaharan Africa: This region remains the most heavily affected by HIV/AIDS, with nearly two-thirds of all HIV infections occurring here. In some countries, the prevalence rate among adults is extremely high.

Asia and the Pacific: This region has the second-largest number of people living with HIV. Key populations, such as sex workers and injecting drug users, are at higher risk.

Eastern Europe and Central Asia: The number of new infections has been on the rise in this region due to injecting drug use and limited access to prevention and treatment.

Latin America: The epidemic varies widely across countries in this region, with concentrated epidemics among certain populations, such as men who have sex with men and transgender individuals.

- **Social and Economic Impact**:

Loss of Lives: Since the beginning of the epidemic, over 36 million people have died from AIDS-related illnesses. HIV/AIDS has claimed more lives than any other infectious disease in human history.

Economic Consequences: The epidemic places a significant economic burden on individuals, families, and healthcare systems. Productivity losses due to illness and death have widespread economic implications.

- **Social Stigma and Discrimination**:

HIV/AIDS has been accompanied by considerable stigma and discrimination, which can have detrimental effects on individuals and communities. Fear of discrimination often deters people from getting tested and seeking treatment.

Discrimination against key affected populations, such as LGBTQ+ individuals and sex workers, exacerbates the epidemic among these groups.

- **Healthcare System**:

HIV/AIDS places a considerable strain on healthcare systems, particularly in resource-limited settings. Access to antiretroviral therapy (ART) is critical for those living with HIV, but not everyone has equal access to these life saving medications.

The HIV epidemic has led to the development of specialized clinics, treatment centers, and services dedicated to HIV care.

- **Global Response**:

The global response to HIV/AIDS has been multifaceted and collaborative. International organizations, governments, NGOs, and activists have played crucial roles in raising awareness, providing resources, and advocating for policies that address the epidemic.

The United Nations established UNAIDS to coordinate global efforts to combat HIV/AIDS.

In conclusion, HIV/AIDS is a complex and enduring global health challenge that continues to affect millions of lives worldwide. While there have been significant advances in prevention, treatment, and awareness, the epidemic persists, and challenges such as stigma, discrimination, and access to healthcare persist. A continued commitment to comprehensive prevention strategies, widespread testing, improved treatment access, and destigmatization efforts are essential to reducing the impact of HIV/AIDS and ultimately achieving the goal of an AIDS-free generation.

The Importance of HIV Prevention and Awareness:

HIV (Human Immunodeficiency Virus) prevention and awareness are paramount in the global effort to combat the HIV/AIDS epidemic. These initiatives play a crucial role in reducing new infections, improving the quality of life for those living with HIV, and ultimately working towards the goal of ending the epidemic.

Here's why HIV prevention and awareness are of utmost importance:

Saving Lives:

HIV is a life-threatening virus that, if left untreated, can progress to AIDS (Acquired Immunodeficiency Syndrome), making the body vulnerable to opportunistic infections and cancers. Prevention measures save lives by reducing the number of new infections.

Reducing Transmission:

Awareness campaigns educate individuals about how HIV is transmitted and how to protect themselves and others. Promoting safe practices like condom use, regular testing, and harm reduction strategies among at-risk populations significantly reduces the risk of transmission.

Early Detection and Treatment:

HIV awareness encourages regular testing and early diagnosis. Detecting HIV early allows individuals to access lifesaving antiretroviral therapy (ART) promptly. Effective treatment can suppress the virus, slow disease progression, and improve the quality and length of life for those living with HIV.

Combating Stigma and Discrimination:

HIV awareness efforts work to dispel myths and reduce the stigma and discrimination associated with the virus. Reducing stigma encourages people to seek testing, treatment, and support without fear of judgment or discrimination.

Empowering Communities:

Community-based HIV prevention and awareness initiatives empower individuals to take control of their sexual health and make informed decisions. Educated communities are better equipped to protect themselves and their partners.

Protecting vulnerable populations:

Certain populations, such as sex workers, men who have sex with men, transgender individuals, and injecting drug users, are at higher risk of HIV infection. Tailored prevention and awareness programs are essential to address their unique needs and challenges.

Preventing Mother-to-Child Transmission:

Awareness and prevention efforts include programs to prevent mother-to-child transmission of HIV. With appropriate interventions, the risk of transmitting the virus from an HIV-positive mother to her child can be greatly reduced.

Global Health Security:

HIV/AIDS has significant public health and economic implications. Preventing new infections and reducing the impact of the epidemic contribute to global health security by preventing health system overloads and safeguarding economic stability.

International Collaboration:

HIV/AIDS is a global issue, and international collaboration is essential. Awareness campaigns and prevention efforts facilitate cooperation between countries, organizations, and individuals working towards a common goal.

Research and Development:

HIV prevention and awareness efforts often support research into new prevention methods, treatments, and potential vaccines. Advancements in these areas are critical to the long-term fight against the virus.

In conclusion, HIV prevention and awareness are vital components of the strategy to control and ultimately end the HIV/AIDS epidemic. These efforts save lives, reduce transmission, combat stigma, and empower communities to protect themselves. A global commitment to comprehensive prevention strategies, widespread testing, destigmatization, and improved treatment access is essential in the ongoing battle against HIV/AIDS.

CHAPTER 2: UNDERSTANDING HIV/AIDS

HIV (Human Immunodeficiency Virus) and AIDS (Acquired Immunodeficiency Syndrome) are two closely related yet distinct conditions that have had a profound impact on public health. To fully grasp the significance of HIV/AIDS, it's essential to understand what each term means, how the virus is transmitted, and the risk factors associated with infection.

What is HIV?

HIV is a virus that attacks the immune system, specifically the body's CD4 cells (T cells), which play a crucial role in fighting infections. Over time, if left untreated, HIV can severely damage the immune system, making it difficult for the body to fight off infections and diseases.

There are two main types of HIV

HIV-1 is the most common and widespread strain of the virus.

HIV2 is less common and primarily found in West Africa.

HIV infection progresses through stages

Acute HIV Infection: The initial stage, often characterized by flu-like symptoms, occurs within a few weeks of exposure.

Chronic HIV Infection: During this stage, the virus continues to replicate but may not cause noticeable symptoms.

 AIDS is the advanced stage of HIV infection, characterized by severe immune system damage and the development of opportunistic infections and cancers.

What is AIDS?

AIDS is the final stage of HIV infection. It is diagnosed when the immune system becomes severely compromised, as measured by a low CD4 cell count (typically below 200 cells/mm3) or when specific AIDS-defining illnesses occur.

AIDS-defining illnesses include conditions like Kaposi's sarcoma, Pneumocystis pneumonia, and certain types of cancer and fungal infections. When someone with HIV develops one of these illnesses, they are said to have AIDS.

Transmission Methods and Risk Factors

HIV is primarily transmitted through the following methods:

Unprotected Sexual Contact: The most common mode of transmission is through sexual intercourse with an HIV-positive partner without using a condom. Both vaginal and anal sex can transmit the virus.

Sharing Needles: HIV can be spread through sharing needles or syringes contaminated with the blood of an infected person, such as in the case of injecting drug use.

Mother-to-Child Transmission: An HIV-positive mother can transmit the virus to her child during pregnancy, childbirth, or breastfeeding. However, with proper medical care and prevention measures, the risk of transmission can be significantly reduced.

Blood Transfusions and Organ Transplants: In the past, there were cases of HIV transmission through contaminated blood products and organ transplants. However, rigorous screening and testing procedures have greatly minimized this risk.

Occupational Exposure: Healthcare workers may be at risk of HIV transmission if they are accidentally exposed to infected blood, such as through needlestick injuries.

Risk Factors

- Engaging in unprotected sexual activity with multiple partners or with partners of unknown HIV status.
- Sharing needles or syringes for drug use.
- Having another sexually transmitted infection (STI) can increase the risk of HIV transmission.
- Receiving transfusions or organ transplants in areas with inadequate screening procedures.
- Being born to an HIV-positive mother without appropriate medical interventions.

Preventing HIV infection involves practicing safe sex, getting tested and knowing your partner's status, using clean needles for drug use, taking preexposure prophylaxis (PrEP) if at high risk, and receiving antiretroviral therapy (ART) if living with HIV. Education and awareness about these transmission methods and risk factors are essential in reducing the spread of HIV and curbing the AIDS epidemic.

CHAPTER 3: HIV TESTING AND DIAGNOSIS

Testing and diagnosis are critical components of HIV prevention and management. Early detection is particularly important as it allows individuals to access timely treatment and take steps to prevent further transmission.

The importance of early detection

The importance of early detection in the context of various health conditions, including infectious diseases like HIV, cannot be overstated. Early detection has numerous benefits that not only impact individual health but also have broader societal and public health implications.
 Here's why early detection is crucial:

Timely Treatment and Management:
   Early detection allows for the prompt initiation of appropriate treatment and management strategies. In the case of HIV, early diagnosis enables individuals to start antiretroviral therapy (ART) sooner. ART is highly effective

in suppressing the virus, slowing disease progression, and preserving immune function.

Improved Health Outcomes:

Early treatment can help maintain a healthier immune system. People living with HIV who are diagnosed and treated early are less likely to develop opportunistic infections and AIDS-related illnesses, leading to a higher quality of life.

Reduced Transmission Risk:

Individuals who are aware of their HIV positive status and are on effective treatment are significantly less likely to transmit the virus to others. This concept is known as "Undetectable = Untransmittable" (U=U). Early detection and treatment play a vital role in preventing new infections.

Preventing Complications:

In many health conditions, early detection can help prevent or reduce the risk of complications. For instance, early detection of cancer often allows for less aggressive treatments and better outcomes.

Lower Healthcare Costs:

Early detection can lead to less complex and less costly treatments. Preventing the progression of a disease through early detection can save both individuals and healthcare systems significant financial burdens.

Psychological and Emotional Benefits:

Early detection provides individuals with a sense of control and empowerment. Knowing one's health status allows for informed decision-making, reduced anxiety, and better mental wellbeing.

Opportunity for Lifestyle Changes:

In many cases, early detection provides an opportunity to make lifestyle changes that can improve health outcomes. For instance, early detection of diabetes allows individuals to adopt healthier eating habits and exercise routines.

Public Health Impact:

On a broader scale, early detection plays a pivotal role in public health. Identifying cases of infectious diseases early can trigger public health responses to prevent outbreaks and epidemics.

Contact Tracing and Prevention:

In infectious diseases like COVID-19 and sexually transmitted infections like HIV, early detection enables contact tracing efforts. Identifying and notifying potentially exposed individuals helps prevent further transmission.

Research and Development:

Early detection and diagnosis contribute to the advancement of medical research and the development of new treatments and prevention strategies. Researchers rely on early cases to study disease progression and treatment outcomes.

In conclusion, early detection is a cornerstone of effective healthcare. Whether it's HIV, cancer, diabetes, or other health conditions, early diagnosis provides individuals with the best chance for successful treatment and improved overall health. Additionally, it has broader implications for public health, prevention efforts, and medical research. Regular health checkups and screenings are essential components of maintaining one's health and wellbeing.

Different types of HIV tests

There are several different types of HIV tests available, each with its own characteristics, advantages, and considerations.

These tests play a crucial role in diagnosing HIV infection, monitoring disease progression, and guiding treatment decisions.

Here are the main types of HIV tests:

Antibody Tests:

Rapid Antibody Test: This is one of the most common and widely used HIV tests. It detects antibodies produced by the immune system in response to HIV infection. Results are typically available within 20 to 30 minutes. Rapid antibody tests are often used in clinics, hospitals, and community centers for quick screening.

ELISA (Enzyme-Linked Immunosorbent Assay) Test:
ELISA is a laboratory-based test that also detects HIV antibodies. While it provides highly accurate results, it may take a few days to receive the results because the blood sample is sent to a laboratory for analysis.

Nucleic Acid Tests (NATs):
NATs are highly sensitive and specific tests that directly detect the genetic material of the virus, either HIV RNA (ribonucleic acid) or HIV DNA (deoxyribonucleic acid). These tests can detect HIV very early after infection, sometimes within days.

NATs are often used in situations where early detection is crucial, such as for newborns born to HIV-positive mothers or during emergency testing after potential HIV exposure.

AntigenAntibody Tests:

These tests detect both HIV antibodies and antigens (proteins produced by the virus). They are also referred to as fourth-generation tests. Antigen-antibody tests can detect HIV infection earlier than antibody-only tests because they identify the presence of viral antigens during the acute phase of infection.

Western Blot Test:

The Western blot test is a confirmatory test used to verify the results of an initial positive antibody test. It is highly specific but may not be as sensitive as other tests in the early stages of infection.

Home Testing Kits:

Some countries offer FDA-approved home HIV testing kits that allow individuals to test themselves in the privacy of their own homes. These kits typically involve a fingerstick blood sample or oral swab, which is then sent to a laboratory for analysis. Results are often available online or via phone.

Point of Care Tests:

Point-of-care tests are rapid tests that can be administered outside of a traditional laboratory setting. They are often used in outreach programs, mobile clinics, and nonclinical settings. These tests provide quick results, similar to rapid antibody tests.

Self-testing kits:

Self-testing kits allow individuals to collect their own samples, usually through an oral swab, and obtain results at home. They are designed to be user-friendly and are often accompanied by clear instructions.

It's important to note that no single HIV test is 100% accurate at all stages of infection. The choice of test may depend on factors such as the time since potential exposure, the testing location, and specific clinical circumstances. In some cases, additional testing or follow-up may be necessary to confirm the HIV status.

It's also essential to remember that while these tests are powerful tools for diagnosing HIV, they are most effective when used in conjunction with other prevention strategies, such as safe sex practices and harm reduction for at-risk populations. Additionally, pre- and post-test counseling are integral parts of HIV testing to provide support and guidance to individuals.

Where to get tested

Getting tested for HIV is a crucial step in taking control of your sexual health and preventing the spread of the virus. There are various options for where to get tested for HIV, and the choice depends on your preferences, accessibility, and confidentiality needs.

Here are some common places where you can get tested for HIV:

- **Healthcare Providers**:

Primary Care Physicians: Many people choose to get tested for HIV during routine check-ups with their family doctor or general practitioner. Healthcare providers can offer a range of testing options, including rapid antibody tests and laboratory-based tests.

Specialized Clinics: Some healthcare facilities, especially in urban areas, have specialized clinics or departments dedicated to sexual health and HIV testing. These clinics often have staff experienced in HIV care and counseling.

- **Public Health Clinics**:

Local Health Departments: Public health clinics run by local or state health departments frequently offer free or low-cost HIV testing services. These clinics may also provide information about prevention and support services.

- **Community Health Centers**:

Federally Qualified Health Centers (FQHCs) and community health centers provide comprehensive healthcare services, including HIV testing and counseling. They often serve underserved populations and offer sliding-scale fees based on income.

- **HIV Testing Events**:

Community Events: Many communities host periodic HIV testing events, particularly during awareness campaigns like National HIV Testing Day (June 27th). These events may offer free and confidential testing.

Mobile Testing Units: Some organizations operate mobile testing units that travel to various locations, making HIV testing more accessible to different communities.

- **Pharmacies**:

In some regions, pharmacies offer rapid HIV testing services. These tests can provide results in a short period of time and are often available without an appointment. Check with your local pharmacies for availability.

- **Online Services**:

Some online platforms offer home HIV testing kits. Individuals can order these kits, collect their own samples (usually a fingerstick blood sample or oral swab), and send them to a laboratory for analysis. Results are typically delivered online or via phone.

- **College and University Health Centers**:

Many educational institutions have health centers that provide confidential HIV testing services for students and staff. These centers may also offer sexual health education and support.

- **Nonprofit Organizations and AIDS Service Organizations (ASOs)**:

Many nonprofit organizations and ASOs dedicated to HIV/AIDS prevention and support provide testing services. They often offer a range of resources, including counseling, prevention education, and referrals for care.

- **Clinics Specializing in LGBTQ+ Health**: LGBTQ+ community centers and clinics may offer HIV testing services tailored to the specific needs and concerns of LGBTQ+ individuals. These clinics are often inclusive and provide a safe space for testing.

- **Private Testing Facilities**: Some private healthcare facilities and laboratories offer confidential HIV testing services. These facilities may provide a range of testing options, including rapid tests and more comprehensive panels.

When choosing where to get tested, consider factors such as convenience, confidentiality, cost, and the type of test you prefer. It's important to remember that HIV testing is typically confidential, and healthcare providers and testing centers adhere to strict privacy guidelines. Regardless of where you choose to get tested, remember that knowing your HIV status is a responsible and proactive step in managing your sexual health and preventing further transmission of the virus.

CHAPTER 4: PREVENTION STRATEGIES

HIV prevention strategies are essential in reducing the spread of the virus and protecting individuals from infection. These strategies encompass a range of approaches, including behavioral measures, biomedical interventions, and public health initiatives.

Abstinence and Safer Sex Practices

Abstinence and safer sex practices are fundamental components of HIV prevention and sexual health. These strategies are essential for reducing the risk of HIV transmission and the spread of other sexually transmitted infections (STIs).

Here's a closer look at abstinence and safer sex practices:

- **Abstinence**:

Abstinence refers to the choice to abstain from sexual activity, including vaginal, anal, or oral intercourse. It is considered one of the most effective methods of preventing HIV and STIs because it eliminates the risk of sexual transmission entirely.

Here are some key points about abstinence:

Effectiveness: Abstinence is 100% effective at preventing HIV and STIs when consistently practiced.

Personal Choice: Abstinence is a personal choice and can be influenced by cultural, religious, emotional, or individual reasons. People of all ages may choose abstinence at different points in their lives.

Education and Support: Comprehensive sex education programs often include information about abstinence as one of the choices available to individuals. It's important to provide education and support for those who choose abstinence to make informed decisions about their sexual health.

- **Safer Sex Practices:**

Safer sex practices are essential for individuals who are sexually active and may have multiple partners or engage in sexual activities that carry a risk of HIV and STI transmission. These practices reduce the risk of infection while allowing individuals to maintain a healthy and active sexual life. Key safer sex practices include:

Condom Use: Consistently and correctly using latex or polyurethane condoms during sexual intercourse (vaginal, anal, or oral) is highly effective at preventing HIV and many other STIs. Condoms create a barrier that prevents contact between bodily fluids, reducing the risk of transmission.

Regular Testing: Getting tested for HIV and other STIs regularly is an essential part of safer sex practices. Knowing your own status and that of your partner(s) allows for informed decision-making about sexual health.

Limiting Sexual Partners: Reducing the number of sexual partners can lower the risk of exposure to HIV and STIs. Having a mutually monogamous, long-term relationship with an HIV-negative partner is a safer sex practice.

Preventing Mother-to-Child Transmission: Pregnant women living with HIV can reduce the risk of transmitting the virus to their infants through medical interventions, including taking antiretroviral medications during pregnancy, childbirth, and breastfeeding.

Safe Injection Practices: For individuals who inject drugs, using sterile needles and syringes and avoiding needle sharing is crucial to preventing HIV transmission among this population.

Dental Dams and Latex Gloves: For oral sex and manual stimulation, dental dams and latex gloves can be used as barriers to reduce the risk of HIV and STI transmission.

Pre Exposure Prophylaxis (PrEP): PrEP is an effective prevention method for individuals at high risk of HIV infection. It involves taking a daily pill containing antiretroviral drugs to reduce the risk of contracting HIV.

Post Exposure Prophylaxis (PEP): PEP is a time-limited course of antiretroviral medications taken after potential exposure to HIV. It is intended to prevent HIV infection when started within 72 hours (ideally within 24 hours) of a high-risk exposure.

Safer sex practices empower individuals to take control of their sexual health and reduce the risk of HIV and STI transmission. Open and honest communication with sexual partners, regular testing, and access to prevention methods are essential components of practicing safer sex.

Use of condoms and barriers

The use of condoms and barriers is a highly effective strategy for preventing the transmission of HIV and other sexually transmitted infections (STIs). Condoms and other barrier methods create a physical barrier between sexual partners, preventing the exchange of bodily fluids and reducing the risk of infection.

Here's a closer look at the use of condoms and barriers to HIV and STI prevention:

1. **Condoms**:

Latex and Polyurethane Condoms: Condoms are sheaths made of latex or polyurethane that are worn over the penis during sexual intercourse. They are one of the most accessible and widely used methods of protection against HIV and STIs.

Effectiveness: When used consistently and correctly, condoms are highly effective at preventing the transmission of HIV and many other STIs, including gonorrhea, chlamydia, and syphilis. They provide a physical barrier that blocks the exchange of semen, vaginal fluids, and blood, all of which can carry infectious agents.

Types of condoms:

Male condoms: Worn over the penis, male condoms are available in various sizes and types, including latex, polyurethane, and lambskin (though lambskin condoms may not provide protection against HIV and other smaller viruses).

Female Condoms: Female condoms are worn inside the vagina and provide protection for both partners. They are made of polyurethane and can be inserted up to eight hours before intercourse.

Condoms and Lubrication: Using water- or silicone-based lubricants with condoms can reduce friction, enhance comfort, and prevent condom breakage. However, it's essential to avoid oil-based lubricants (e.g., petroleum jelly), as they can weaken latex condoms.

Consistency and Correct Use: For condoms to be effective, they must be used consistently and correctly during every sexual encounter. This includes checking for proper storage and expiration dates and ensuring the condom is unrolled onto the erect penis with no air trapped inside.

2. **Dental Dams and Latex Gloves**:

Dental Dams: Dental dams are thin, flexible sheets made of latex or polyurethane. They are used as a barrier during oral sex, providing protection when placed over the genital or anal area. Dental dams prevent direct contact with bodily fluids, reducing the risk of HIV and STI transmission.

Latex Gloves: Latex gloves are often used during manual stimulation, such as fingering or fisting, to prevent skin-to-skin contact and potential exposure to blood or bodily fluids. They are an important tool for reducing the risk of transmission.

3. **Effectiveness and Considerations**:

Barrier methods are most effective when used consistently and correctly during sexual activities that carry a risk of HIV and STI transmission.

They are essential for individuals who engage in sexual activities with multiple partners, those in serodiscordant relationships (where one partner is HIVpositive and the other is HIVnegative), and anyone who wants to reduce their risk of infection.

While condoms and barriers are highly effective, no prevention method is 100% foolproof. It's essential to combine barrier methods with regular HIV and STI testing, communication with sexual partners, and other prevention strategies like PrEP (pre-exposure prophylaxis) for those at high risk.

Barrier methods are important tools for promoting sexual health and reducing the spread of HIV and STIs. Individuals should be informed about these methods, have access to them, and be encouraged to use them consistently to protect themselves and their sexual partners. Open and honest communication about sexual health and prevention methods is crucial to maintaining safe and satisfying sexual relationships.

Pre-exposure prophylaxis (PrEP) and post-exposure prophylaxis (PEP)

Pre Exposure prophylaxis (PrEP) and postexposure prophylaxis (PEP) are two critical biomedical interventions in the prevention of HIV infection. These medications are used to reduce the risk of contracting HIV before and after potential exposure.

Here's an overview of PrEP and PEP:

Pre-Exposure Prophylaxis (PrEP):

What is PrEP? PrEP is a preventive strategy for individuals at high risk of HIV infection. It involves taking a daily oral medication that contains a combination of antiretroviral drugs. The goal of PrEP is to provide a protective shield against HIV before potential exposure occurs.

Who Should Consider PrEP? PrEP is recommended for individuals at increased risk of HIV infection, including:

1. Men who have sex with men (MSM) and engage in condomless anal sex
2. Heterosexual individuals with partners known to have HIV or engage in behaviors that increase the risk of HIV transmission
3. People who inject drugs and share needles or drug equipment
4. Individuals in serodiscordant relationships, where one partner is HIV positive and the other is HIV negative,
5. Sex workers and clients in areas with high HIV prevalence

Effectiveness of PrEP:
When taken as prescribed, PrEP is highly effective in preventing HIV infection. Studies have shown that consistent use of PrEP can reduce the risk of HIV transmission by over 90%.
It's essential to take PrEP daily, as prescribed, to maintain protection.

Monitoring and Adherence:
Regular medical checkups and HIV testing are part of PrEP monitoring to ensure that individuals remain HIV-negative. Adherence to the daily medication schedule is critical for PrEP to be effective. Healthcare providers can provide support and guidance on adherence strategies.

Post Exposure Prophylaxis (PEP):

What is PEP? PEP is a time-limited course of antiretroviral medications taken after potential exposure to HIV. It is intended to prevent HIV infection when initiated as soon as possible, ideally within 24 hours, and no later than 72 hours after a high-risk exposure.

When is PEP used? PEP is used in situations where there has been a high-risk exposure to HIV, such as:

1. Unprotected sexual intercourse with a partner known to be HIV positive or of unknown HIV status
2. Occupational exposure, such as needlestick injuries or exposure to potentially HIV-infected blood or bodily fluids in healthcare settings.
3. nonoccupational exposure, such as sexual assault or other situations where potential HIV exposure has occurred.

Effectiveness of PEP:
 PEP is highly effective at preventing HIV infection when started promptly after a high-risk exposure.
 The sooner PEP is initiated, the higher the chances of preventing HIV transmission.

PEP Regimen:
 PEP typically involves taking a combination of antiretroviral drugs for 28 days. The specific medications and duration may vary based on individual circumstances and the source of potential exposure.

Accessing PrEP and PEP:

PrEP and PEP are available through healthcare providers, clinics, and emergency rooms.
Access may vary by region, but guidelines and recommendations are established to ensure that individuals at risk have access to these prevention strategies.

Both PrEP and PEP are valuable tools in a comprehensive approach to preventing HIV infection. They offer options for individuals to protect themselves before and after potential exposure to the virus. However, it's essential to use these medications as part of a broader prevention strategy that includes safer sex practices, regular HIV testing, and open communication with healthcare providers about sexual health.

CHAPTER 5: TREATMENT AND MEDICATIONS

Treatment and medications for HIV have advanced significantly over the years, transforming HIV from a once-fatal disease into a chronic, manageable condition. The primary approach to HIV treatment involves the use of antiretroviral therapy (ART).

Antiretroviral therapy (ART)

Antiretroviral therapy (ART) is a cornerstone in the treatment of HIV (human immunodeficiency virus) infection. This therapeutic approach involves the use of a combination of antiretroviral drugs to suppress the replication of the virus, slow down the progression of the disease, and preserve the immune function of the individual. ART has been a groundbreaking advancement in HIV care, transforming what was once a life threatening illness into a manageable chronic condition.

Here are key aspects of antiretroviral therapy (ART):

Objective of ART:

The primary goal of ART is to achieve and maintain an undetectable viral load in the blood. An undetectable viral load means that the amount of HIV in the bloodstream is so low that it cannot be detected by standard tests. This is associated with improved health outcomes and a significantly reduced risk of transmitting the virus to others.

Classes of antiretroviral Drugs:

- **Nucleoside Reverse Transcriptase Inhibitors (NRTIs)**: These drugs interfere with the reverse transcriptase enzyme, preventing the conversion of viral RNA into DNA.

- **Non-Nucleoside Reverse Transcriptase Inhibitors (NNRTIs)**: These drugs bind to and inhibit the reverse transcriptase enzyme, disrupting the viral replication process.

- **Protease inhibitors (PIs)**: PIs block the activity of the protease enzyme, which is essential for the final stages of viral maturation.

- **Integrase Strand Transfer Inhibitors (INSTIs):** INSTIs block the action of integrase, an enzyme that allows the viral DNA to integrate into the host cell's DNA.

The combination of drugs from different classes is often referred to as highly active antiretroviral therapy (HAART) or combination antiretroviral therapy (cART). This approach is designed to target the virus at multiple stages of its life cycle, reducing the likelihood of developing drug-resistant strains.

Initiation of ART:

The decision to start ART is based on various factors, including the individual's CD4 cell count (a marker of immune function), viral load, overall health, and readiness to adhere to the treatment plan.

Modern guidelines often recommend initiating ART soon after diagnosis, regardless of CD4 count, to achieve better health outcomes and reduce the risk of transmission.

Adherence to Treatment:

Adherence to the prescribed ART regimen is crucial for its effectiveness. Missing doses or not taking the medications consistently can lead to the development of drug-resistant strains of HIV and treatment failure.

Healthcare providers work closely with individuals on ART to support adherence, address any concerns or side effects, and adjust the treatment plan when needed.

Monitoring and Side Effects:

Regular monitoring is essential to assess the individual's response to treatment. This includes measuring CD4 cell counts, viral load, and other relevant markers.

While modern ART regimens are generally well tolerated, some individuals may experience side effects. Common side effects include nausea, fatigue, and changes in lipid levels. Serious side effects are rare but can occur.

Lifespan and Quality of Life:

Effective ART has transformed HIV into a chronic, manageable condition. With proper treatment and care, individuals with HIV can lead healthy and productive lives.

The life expectancy of people with HIV who are on successful ART is approaching that of the general population.

Preventive Impact:

Beyond its therapeutic role, ART is a powerful tool for preventing the transmission of HIV. Individuals with an undetectable viral load are highly unlikely to transmit the virus to their sexual partners, a concept known as "undetectable = untransmittable" (U=U).

Antiretroviral therapy has been a game changer in the field of HIV care, demonstrating the effectiveness of combining multiple drugs to control the virus and improve the health and wellbeing of individuals living with HIV. Ongoing research and development continue to explore new drug classes, formulations, and treatment strategies to further enhance the effectiveness and accessibility of ART.

Managing HIV as a chronic condition

Managing HIV as a chronic condition has become a reality due to significant advancements in medical science and the widespread use of antiretroviral therapy (ART). Here are key aspects of managing HIV as a chronic condition:

- **Antiretroviral Therapy (ART)**:

Initiation of Treatment: Early initiation of ART is a crucial step in managing HIV as a chronic condition. Treatment is often started soon after diagnosis, regardless of CD4 cell count, to achieve optimal health outcomes and reduce the risk of disease progression.

Suppressing Viral Load: The primary goal of ART is to suppress the viral load to undetectable levels. An undetectable viral load means that the amount of HIV in the blood is so low that it cannot be detected by standard tests. This not only improves the individual's health but also greatly reduces the risk of transmitting the virus to others.

Combination Therapy: ART typically involves a combination of antiretroviral drugs from different classes. This approach, often referred to as highly active antiretroviral therapy (HAART), targets the virus at multiple stages of its life cycle, reducing the likelihood of developing drug-resistant strains.

- **Regular medical monitoring**:

CD4 Cell Counts and Viral Load Testing: Regular monitoring of CD4 cell counts and viral load helps healthcare providers assess the immune function and effectiveness of ART. The goal is to maintain a high CD4 count and an undetectable viral load.

Screening for Opportunistic Infections: Individuals with HIV are monitored for opportunistic infections and other HIV-related complications. Early detection and treatment of these conditions contribute to overall health.

Routine Health Checkups: Regular checkups address general health concerns, monitor for potential side effects of medications, and assess overall wellbeing.

- **Adherence to Treatment**:

Importance of Adherence: Adherence to the prescribed ART regimen is critical for its effectiveness. Consistent and correct use of medications helps maintain viral suppression and prevent the development of drug-resistant strains.

Support and Education: Healthcare providers offer support and education to help individuals understand the importance of adherence, manage side effects, and address any concerns related to their treatment plan.

- **Preventive Measures**:

Preventing Transmission (U=U): Individuals with an undetectable viral load due to effective ART are highly unlikely to transmit the virus to their sexual partners. This concept is known as "undetectable = untransmittable" (U=U).

Pre Exposure Prophylaxis (PrEP): In certain circumstances, individuals at high risk of HIV may use PrEP, which involves taking antiretroviral medications to prevent infection.

- **Coordinated Healthcare**:

Multidisciplinary Care: Managing HIV as a chronic condition often involves a multidisciplinary healthcare team, including infectious disease specialists, primary care physicians, nurses, mental health professionals, and social workers.

Addressing Mental Health: Mental health is a crucial aspect of overall wellbeing. Healthcare providers offer support and resources to address any psychological or emotional challenges associated with living with HIV.

- **Lifestyle Factors:**

Healthy Living: Adopting a healthy lifestyle, including regular exercise, a balanced diet, and avoiding substances like tobacco and excessive alcohol, contributes to overall health.

Sexual Health: Open communication with healthcare providers about sexual health, including safe practices and preventive measures, is essential.

- **Long-Term Outcomes:**

Life Expectancy: With effective ART and proper management, individuals with HIV can expect near-normal life expectancies.

Quality of Life: Advances in treatment have improved the quality of life for individuals living with HIV. Many are able to pursue their personal and professional goals with the right medical care and support.

Managing HIV as a chronic condition requires a comprehensive and individualized approach. Regular engagement with healthcare providers, adherence to treatment and preventive measures, and addressing overall wellbeing contribute to successful long-term management. As research continues and new developments emerge, the outlook for individuals living with HIV continues to improve.

The role of healthcare providers

The role of healthcare providers is crucial to the comprehensive care and management of individuals living with HIV. Healthcare professionals play multifaceted roles that span diagnosis, treatment, prevention, and support. key aspects of the role of healthcare providers in HIV care:

- **Diagnosis and Counseling:**

Testing and Diagnosis: Healthcare providers are responsible for conducting HIV tests, interpreting results, and delivering a diagnosis to individuals. This process involves providing information about the virus, the implications of the diagnosis, and initiating discussions about the next steps.

Counseling and Support: Offering emotional support and counseling is an integral part of the diagnostic process. Healthcare providers guide individuals through the initial shock of diagnosis, address concerns, and provide information about living with HIV.

- **Treatment Initiation and Monitoring**:

ART Initiation: Healthcare providers are responsible for determining when to initiate antiretroviral therapy (ART). This decision is based on factors such as CD4 cell counts, viral load, and the overall health of the individual.

Treatment Monitoring: Regular monitoring involves assessing the effectiveness of ART through tests like CD4 cell counts and viral load measurements. Healthcare providers use this information to adjust treatment plans as needed.

Adherence Support: Ensuring that individuals adhere to their prescribed treatment regimen is vital for the success of

ART. Healthcare providers provide education, support, and strategies to enhance adherence.

- **Preventive Measures**:

PrEP and PEP: Healthcare providers educate individuals at high risk of HIV about preexposure prophylaxis (PrEP) and postexposure prophylaxis (PEP). They prescribe and monitor the use of these preventive medications.

Promoting Safer Practices: Providers discuss and promote safer sex practices, including condom use, to prevent the transmission of HIV and other sexually transmitted infections.

- **Managing coexisting conditions**:

Multidisciplinary Care: Many individuals with HIV may have coexisting conditions or comorbidities. Healthcare providers coordinate with specialists in areas such as cardiology, dermatology, and mental health to provide comprehensive care.

Addressing mental health: HIV can have significant mental health implications. Healthcare providers, including psychologists and social workers, offer support and counseling to address mental health challenges.

- **Regular Checkups and Screenings**:

Routine Health Assessments: Regular checkups are essential for monitoring overall health. Healthcare providers conduct routine physical examinations, screenings for opportunistic infections, and assessments of medication side effects.

Vaccinations: Ensuring that individuals receive necessary vaccinations is part of preventive care. Healthcare providers may administer vaccines for conditions such as influenza and pneumonia.

- **Educating and Empowering**:

Health Education: Healthcare providers offer ongoing health education to individuals living with HIV. This includes information about their condition, treatment options, and strategies for maintaining overall wellbeing.

Empowering Decision-Making: Encouraging active participation in healthcare decision-making empowers individuals to take control of their health. Informed decision-making contributes to better adherence to treatment plans.

- **Community Engagement and Advocacy**:

Community Resources: Healthcare providers connect individuals with community resources, support groups, and advocacy organizations that can provide additional support.

Advocacy for Access to Care: Providers advocate for policies and practices that enhance access to healthcare services and reduce stigma and discrimination against individuals living with HIV.

- **Crisis Intervention and Support**:

Crisis Management: In situations of medical crises or emergencies, healthcare providers are at the forefront of managing and stabilizing the individual's health.

Psychosocial Support: Beyond medical care, providers offer psychosocial support to help individuals cope with challenges and maintain a positive outlook.

The role of healthcare providers in HIV care is dynamic and extends beyond medical interventions. It encompasses emotional support, education, prevention, and advocacy. Collaborative and patient-centered care is key to achieving successful long-term management of HIV and promoting the overall wellbeing of individuals living with the virus.

CHAPTER 6: STIGMA AND DISCRIMINATION

Stigma and discrimination related to HIV/AIDS have been significant barriers in the global response to the epidemic. Understanding, combating, and addressing HIV-related stigma is crucial for creating supportive environments, improving public health outcomes, and ensuring the wellbeing of individuals living with HIV.

Understanding and combating HIV-related stigma

Understanding and combating HIV-related stigma is crucial for improving the quality of life for individuals living with HIV (Human Immunodeficiency Virus) and promoting a more inclusive and supportive society. Stigma associated with HIV is often rooted in fear, ignorance, and misconceptions about the virus. Addressing these issues requires a multifaceted approach that includes education, awareness, and advocacy. Here are key aspects of understanding and combating HIV-related stigma:

Understanding HIV-related stigma:

Definition: Stigma is a set of negative beliefs, attitudes, and behaviors directed at people perceived to have a particular characteristic or condition, in this case, HIV infection.

- **Forms of stigma**:

Public stigma: negative attitudes and discriminatory behaviors from the general population

Self-stigma: internalized shame or negative self-perception experienced by individuals living with HIV

Enacted stigma: discriminatory actions directed at individuals based on their HIV status.

- **Root causes**:

Misinformation: lack of accurate knowledge about how HIV is transmitted and prevented.

Fear of Contagion: Unfounded fears about casual transmission of the virus

Stigmatizing Beliefs: Moral judgments and stereotypes associated with the modes of transmission

- **Impact on Individuals:**

Delayed Testing and Treatment Fear of stigma can discourage people from getting tested for HIV or seeking treatment.

Isolation and Discrimination: Stigmatizing attitudes may lead to social isolation, discrimination, and loss of support systems.

Mental Health Consequences: Stigma is linked to increased rates of anxiety, depression, and lower overall mental wellbeing among individuals living with HIV.

- **Combating HIV-related Stigma:**

Education and Awareness:
Community education: promoting accurate information about HIV transmission and prevention
School Programs: Including comprehensive sex education in schools to dispel myths and reduce stigma
Media Campaigns: Utilizing mass media to disseminate factual information and challenge stigmatizing narratives

- **Humanizing the Experience:**

Personal Stories: Sharing personal narratives of individuals living with HIV to humanize the experience and challenge stereotypes

Faces of HIV Campaigns: Featuring diverse faces and stories to counteract stigmatizing images

- **Community Engagement:**

Support Groups: Establishing and promoting support groups for individuals living with HIV to share experiences and provide mutual support

Community Dialogues: Creating safe spaces for open discussions about HIV to challenge stigma

- **Anti Stigma Programs:**

Training Healthcare Providers: Ensuring that healthcare professionals are trained to provide nonjudgmental and supportive care

Workplace Anti Stigma Programs: Encouraging businesses and organizations to create environments free of discrimination

- **Legal protections:**

Advocacy for Legal Reforms: Working towards legal protections that prevent discrimination based on HIV status

Challenging Stigmatizing Laws: Advocating for the repeal of laws that criminalize HIV transmission

- **Peer-led Initiatives:**

Peer Educators: Training individuals living with HIV as peer educators to provide support, information, and combat stigma

Peer Led Support Groups: Establishing peer led support groups to create a sense of community and shared experience

- **Intersectionality and Cultural Competence:**

Recognizing Diversity: Acknowledging that stigma affects different communities differently and tailoring interventions accordingly

Cultural Competence Training: Ensuring that interventions are culturally sensitive and respectful of diverse identities

- **Promoting U=U (Undetectable = untransmittable):**

Publicizing Scientific Evidence: Promoting the fact that individuals with an undetectable viral load cannot transmit HIV to their partners This challenges the fear of contagion.

- **Ongoing Challenges and Future Directions**:

Continued Advocacy: Advocacy efforts must continue to challenge stigma at societal, institutional, and individual levels.

Global Cooperation: International collaboration is essential to share best practices and develop strategies for combating stigma on a global scale.

In conclusion, understanding and combating HIV-related stigma require a comprehensive approach that involves education, community engagement, legal advocacy, and the promotion of empathy and understanding. By addressing the root causes of stigma and fostering a more inclusive society, it is possible to create an environment where individuals living with HIV can access the support and care they need without fear of discrimination or judgment.

Legal protections and advocacy efforts

Legal protections and advocacy efforts play a crucial role in addressing HIV-related stigma and discrimination. While progress has been made, many individuals living with HIV (Human Immunodeficiency Virus) still face legal challenges that can impact their rights, access to healthcare, and overall well being. Legal protections and advocacy efforts are essential in creating an environment that is supportive, nondiscriminatory, and inclusive.
Here are key aspects of legal protections and advocacy efforts related to HIV:

- **Legal protections**:

Anti Discrimination Laws: Many countries and regions have enacted laws that explicitly prohibit discrimination on the basis of HIV status. These laws may extend to various aspects of life, including employment, housing, education, and healthcare.

Privacy and Confidentiality Laws: Laws protecting the privacy of individuals' medical information, including their HIV status, are critical for safeguarding against unauthorized disclosure.

Criminalization Reform: Some jurisdictions have moved towards reforming laws that criminalize HIV transmission. Such laws often perpetuate stigma and may result in unjust prosecutions.

Healthcare Access Laws: Legal protections may be in place to ensure that individuals living with HIV have equal access to healthcare services without facing discrimination from healthcare providers.

Employment Protections: Laws may prohibit discrimination against employees based on their HIV status and require employers to make reasonable accommodations.

Legal Gender Recognition: In some regions, legal protections include recognition of gender identity, which is particularly important for transgender individuals, including those living with HIV.

- **Advocacy Efforts:**

Awareness Campaigns: Advocacy groups work to raise awareness about the impact of HIV-related stigma and discrimination. This includes dispelling myths, educating the public, and promoting understanding.

Policy Advocacy: Advocacy organizations engage with policymakers to promote and strengthen legal protections for individuals living with HIV. This may involve pushing for new legislation, amending existing laws, or challenging discriminatory practices.

Community Mobilization: Grassroots advocacy involves mobilizing communities affected by HIV to actively participate in advocating for their rights. This includes training community members to be advocates and providing resources for self-advocacy.

Litigation and Legal Challenges: Advocacy groups may pursue legal action to challenge discriminatory laws, policies, or practices. This could involve filing lawsuits, submitting amicus curiae briefs, or supporting individuals facing legal challenges due to their HIV status.

International Advocacy: Organizations work at the international level to advocate for the rights of individuals living with HIV. This includes engaging with international bodies, such as the United Nations, to shape global policies and guidelines.

Partnerships with Legal Professionals: Advocacy groups often collaborate with legal professionals to provide expertise in crafting legal strategies, interpreting existing laws, and challenging discriminatory practices.

Research and Documentation: Advocacy efforts are strengthened by research documenting instances of discrimination, barriers to healthcare, and the impact of laws and policies on individuals living with HIV.

- **Challenges and Ongoing Work:**

Inconsistent Enforcement: Even when legal protections exist, enforcement may be inconsistent. Advocacy efforts often include holding institutions accountable for implementing and enforcing anti discrimination laws.

Stigmatizing Laws: In some cases, laws themselves may contribute to stigma. Advocacy work includes challenging and reforming laws that perpetuate discrimination and hinder public health efforts.

Intersectionality: Advocacy must recognize and address the intersectionality of discrimination, considering how factors such as race, gender, sexual orientation, and socioeconomic status intersect with HIV-related stigma.

Global Advocacy: Since HIV is a global issue, advocacy efforts often extend beyond national borders. Organizations work collaboratively to address global challenges, share best practices, and advocate for international standards.

In conclusion, legal protections and advocacy efforts are essential components of the broader strategy to combat HIV-related stigma and discrimination. By working to create and strengthen legal frameworks that protect the rights of individuals living with HIV and by advocating for broader societal change, organizations and advocates contribute to fostering environments that are supportive, understanding, and inclusive.

Personal stories of individuals affected by stigma

Personal stories of individuals affected by HIV-related stigma provide powerful insights into the real-life impact of discrimination and prejudice. These narratives humanize the experiences of those living with HIV, shedding light on the challenges they face as well as their resilience and strength. Sharing personal stories is a crucial tool in advocacy efforts, fostering empathy, understanding, and encouraging societal change.

Here are key aspects of the personal stories of individuals affected by HIV-related stigma:

1. Humanizing the Experience:

Breaking Stereotypes: Personal stories challenge stereotypes and misconceptions about HIV. They illustrate that individuals living with the virus are diverse and come from all walks of life.

Putting a Face to the Issue: Personal narratives put a human face to the statistics, helping people see beyond the label of "HIV positive" and recognize the shared humanity.

Emotional Impact: Hearing personal stories can evoke empathy and emotional connection, fostering a deeper understanding of the challenges faced by individuals living with HIV.

2. Challenges Faced by Individuals:

Stigma and Discrimination: Personal stories often highlight instances of stigma and discrimination faced by individuals living with HIV in various aspects of their lives, including healthcare, employment, and social interactions.

Impact on Mental Health: Narratives may discuss the emotional toll of stigma, revealing the impact on mental health, self-esteem, and overall well being.

Isolation and Fear of Disclosure: Many individuals living with HIV experience isolation due to fear of disclosure. Personal stories shed light on the internal struggles faced when deciding whether to share their HIV status.

3. Resilience and Empowerment:

Overcoming Adversity: Personal stories often showcase the resilience of individuals who, despite facing stigma, discrimination, and personal challenges, continue to live fulfilling lives.

Advocacy and Empowerment: Some individuals turn their experiences into a source of advocacy, actively working to challenge stigma, raise awareness, and improve the lives of others.

Community Support: Narratives may highlight the importance of community support, whether from friends, family, or support groups, in helping individuals cope with the challenges of living with HIV.

4. Encouraging Dialogue and Understanding:

Open Conversations: Personal stories create opportunities for open and honest conversations about HIV. They encourage dialogue around the importance of reducing stigma and discrimination.

Educational Value: Sharing personal stories contributes to public education by providing real-world examples of the impact of stigma and the importance of empathy and compassion.

Reducing Fear and Misconceptions: Narratives help dispel myths and misconceptions about HIV, addressing fear and ignorance that often contribute to stigma.

5. Intersectionality and Diverse Experiences:

Recognizing Diversity: Personal stories reflect the diversity within the HIV-affected community, acknowledging that experiences of stigma may vary based on factors such as race, gender, sexual orientation, and socioeconomic status.

Intersectional Stigma: Some narratives may explore how intersecting identities contribute to unique experiences of stigma, emphasizing the need for approaches that consider multiple dimensions of discrimination.

6. Media and Storytelling Platforms:

Documentaries and Films: Visual storytelling through documentaries and films can be a powerful medium for sharing personal stories and reaching a wider audience.

Books and Literature: Memoirs and literature written by individuals living with HIV offer in-depth perspectives on their journeys, struggles, and triumphs.

Digital Platforms and Social Media: Blogs, vlogs, and social media platforms provide spaces for individuals to share their stories directly with a global audience.

In conclusion, personal stories of individuals affected by HIV-related stigma are invaluable in the fight against discrimination. By amplifying these narratives, society can foster empathy, challenge stereotypes, and work toward creating environments that are supportive, understanding, and inclusive for individuals living with HIV.

CHAPTER 7: HIV AND VULNERABLE POPULATIONS

HIV/AIDS affects diverse populations around the world, and certain groups are more vulnerable to infection due to various social, economic, and structural factors. Understanding and addressing the specific needs of vulnerable populations is crucial to the global response to HIV/AIDS.

HIV in the LGBTQ+ community

HIV/AIDS has had a significant impact on the LGBTQ+ (Lesbian, Gay, Bisexual, Transgender, and Queer/Questioning) community. While progress has been made in terms of prevention and treatment, certain factors make individuals within the LGBTQ+ community more vulnerable to HIV infection. Understanding these factors and implementing targeted strategies is essential to addressing the unique challenges faced by this community.

- **Higher Prevalence Rates:**

Men who have sex with men (MSM): Globally, MSM have consistently been identified as a high-risk group for HIV transmission. This population is more likely to be exposed to the virus due to various factors, including a higher prevalence within the community.

Transgender Individuals: Studies also indicate elevated rates of HIV infection among transgender individuals, especially transgender women.

- **Stigma and Discrimination:**

Internalized Stigma: LGBTQ+ individuals may face internalized stigma related to their sexual orientation or gender identity, which can impact their self-esteem and mental health.

Societal Stigma: Widespread societal stigma and discrimination can create barriers to accessing HIV prevention, testing, and treatment services. Fear of discrimination may discourage individuals from seeking help.

- **Sexual Health Practices and Risk Factors:**

Condom Use and Risky Behaviors: Factors such as inconsistent condom use, a higher number of sexual partners, and engaging in anal sex without protection contribute to the increased risk of HIV transmission within the LGBTQ+ community.

Substance Use: Substance use, particularly in social settings, may contribute to risky sexual behaviors, further increasing the likelihood of HIV transmission.

- **Mental Health Impact:**

Higher Rates of Mental Health Issues: LGBTQ+ individuals may experience higher rates of mental health issues, including depression and anxiety. Mental health challenges can impact adherence to HIV treatment and overall well being.

Intersectionality: Intersectionality plays a role, with individuals facing compounded challenges when discrimination based on sexual orientation or gender identity intersects with other factors such as race and socioeconomic status.

- **Barriers to Healthcare Access:**

Cultural Competency: Healthcare providers may lack cultural competency in addressing the specific needs of LGBTQ+ individuals. This can create barriers to accessing quality healthcare services, including HIV prevention, testing, and treatment.

Fear of Discrimination: Fear of discrimination within healthcare settings may lead to delayed or avoided healthcare-seeking behavior among LGBTQ+ individuals.

- **Prevention Strategies for the LGBTQ+ Community:**

Comprehensive Sexual Health Education: Implementing comprehensive sexual health education programs that are inclusive of LGBTQ+ experiences can empower individuals to make informed choices.

Increased Access to PrEP: Pre Exposure prophylaxis (PrEP) has proven effective in preventing HIV transmission. Increasing awareness and access to PrEP within the LGBTQ+ community is crucial.

Community Outreach and Testing Programs: Engaging with LGBTQ+ community organizations for outreach and testing programs can help increase awareness and encourage regular testing.

Antistigma Campaigns: Community-led campaigns that challenge stigma and discrimination, both within and outside the LGBTQ+ community, can contribute to creating a more supportive environment.

Healthcare Provider Training: Providing training for healthcare professionals on LGBTQ+ cultural competency can improve healthcare access and reduce discrimination.

Mental Health Support Services: Integrating mental health support services within HIV/AIDS programs can address the mental health challenges faced by LGBTQ+ individuals.

- **Community Empowerment and Advocacy:**

Community Involvement: Engaging the LGBTQ+ community in the design and implementation of HIV prevention and support programs ensures that these initiatives are culturally sensitive and effective.

Advocacy for LGBTQ+ Rights: Advocacy efforts for LGBTQ+ rights, including anti discrimination measures, contribute to creating a more inclusive society and reducing the overall vulnerability of the community.

In conclusion, addressing HIV in the LGBTQ+ community requires a holistic approach that considers the specific challenges faced by individuals within this diverse community. Efforts should focus on reducing stigma, improving access to healthcare, and implementing targeted prevention strategies to create a more supportive environment for LGBTQ+ individuals in the context of HIV/AIDS.

HIV among injection drug users

HIV among injection drug users (IDUs) is a significant public health concern, as the sharing of needles and drug paraphernalia can facilitate the transmission of the virus. Understanding the unique challenges faced by this population is crucial for designing effective prevention and intervention strategies. Here are key aspects related to HIV among injection drug users:

- **High Risk of Transmission**:

Needle Sharing: The primary mode of HIV transmission among injection drug users is through the sharing of needles and syringes contaminated with the virus. This can result in the direct exchange of infected blood.

Increased Vulnerability: The nature of injection drug use increases the risk of blood exposure, making IDUs more susceptible to HIV compared to other populations.

- **Socioeconomic Factors:**

Poverty and Homelessness: Injection drug use is often associated with socioeconomic factors such as poverty and homelessness. Limited access to resources and stable housing can contribute to higher vulnerability.

Limited Healthcare Access: Barriers to healthcare access, including stigma and discrimination, can hinder IDUs from seeking HIV prevention, testing, and treatment services.

- **Stigma and Criminalization**:

Stigmatization of Drug Use: Stigma associated with drug use can lead to the marginalization of IDUs, making them less likely to access healthcare services.

Criminalization of Drug Use: Legal measures that criminalize drug use can exacerbate stigma, leading to fear of legal consequences and reluctance to seek medical assistance.

- **Health Disparities:**

Coinfections: Injection drug users are at an increased risk of coinfections such as Hepatitis C, which can further complicate their health status.

Mental Health Challenges: Substance use disorders often coexist with mental health challenges, and addressing these issues is integral to effective HIV prevention and care.

- **Harm Reduction Strategies:**

Needle Exchange Programs: Providing access to clean needles and syringes through needle exchange programs helps reduce the risk of HIV transmission and other bloodborne infections.

Opioid Substitution Therapy (OST):
Medication-assisted treatments, such as methadone or buprenorphine, can support individuals in reducing or eliminating opioid use, lowering the risk of HIV transmission.

Supervised Injection Facilities: These facilities provide a safe and supervised environment for individuals to inject drugs, reducing the risk of overdose and transmission of infections.

Education and Counseling: Offering educational programs on safe injection practices and providing counseling services can empower IDUs to make informed decisions about their health.

- **Testing and Treatment:**

Regular Testing: Encouraging regular HIV testing among injection drug users is essential for early detection and timely initiation of antiretroviral therapy (ART).

Integrated Care: Integrating HIV testing and treatment services with substance use treatment programs ensures a comprehensive approach to care.

Access to Medication: Ensuring that IDUs have access to HIV medications is critical for their health and for preventing further transmission.

- **Community Engagement and Empowerment:**

Peer Led Interventions: Peer-based programs and outreach initiatives led by individuals with a history of injection drug use can be effective in reaching and supporting the community.

Community Resources: Establishing community resources, including support groups and counseling services, creates a network for individuals to access information and assistance.

Advocacy for Policy Changes: Advocacy efforts can focus on changing policies related to drug use, emphasizing harm reduction, and reducing the criminalization of substance use.

- **Global Perspective:**

International Efforts: Recognizing that injection drug use and HIV transmission are global issues, international collaboration and support are crucial for implementing effective strategies.

In conclusion, addressing HIV among injection drug users requires a comprehensive and compassionate approach that considers the social determinants of health, integrates harm reduction strategies, and engages the community in the design and implementation of interventions. By providing support, reducing stigma, and implementing evidence-based practices, it is possible to make significant strides in preventing HIV transmission among injection drug users and improving their overall health outcomes.

Impact of HIV on women and children

The impact of HIV on women and children is profound, influencing various aspects of their health, social wellbeing, and overall quality of life. The vulnerability of women and children to HIV is shaped by biological, social, and economic factors. Understanding and addressing these impacts are crucial for designing effective strategies for prevention, treatment, and support.

Here are key aspects of the impact of HIV on women and children:

- **Vertical Transmission and Pediatric HIV:**

Mother-to-Child Transmission (MTCT): Without intervention, HIV-positive pregnant women can transmit the virus to their infants during pregnancy, childbirth, or breastfeeding, leading to pediatric HIV infections.

Prevention of MTCT (PMTCT): Implementation of prevention of mother-to-child transmission programs, including antiretroviral therapy (ART) for pregnant women, significantly reduces the risk of vertical transmission.

Early Diagnosis and Treatment: Early diagnosis of pediatric HIV is crucial for initiating timely treatment, improving health outcomes, and preventing the progression to AIDS.

- **Disproportionate Impact on Women**:

Global Burden: Women, particularly in sub-Saharan Africa, bear a disproportionate burden of HIV/AIDS. They account for a significant percentage of new infections and individuals living with HIV in this region.

Biological Vulnerability: Biological factors, including the increased risk of heterosexual transmission, make women more vulnerable to HIV infection.

Gender Inequality: Gender inequalities, including limited decision-making power, economic dependence, and gender-based violence, contribute to women's vulnerability to HIV.

- **Challenges Faced by Women Living with HIV:**

Stigma and Discrimination: Women living with HIV may face stigma and discrimination, impacting their mental health, relationships, and access to healthcare.

Reproductive Health: HIV-positive women may encounter challenges related to reproductive health, family planning, and the fear of transmitting the virus to their partners or children.

Access to Treatment: Barriers to accessing antiretroviral therapy (ART) include socioeconomic factors, stigma, and gender-specific challenges.

- **Impact on Maternal and Child Health:**

Maternal Health: HIV can complicate maternal health, affecting pregnancy outcomes and increasing the risk of maternal mortality, particularly in settings with limited access to healthcare.

Child Health: Children born to HIV-positive mothers may face health challenges, including an increased risk of preterm birth, low birth weight, and potential exposure to the virus during childbirth.

- **Orphanhood and Vulnerability:**

Parental Loss: Children who lose one or both parents to AIDS face challenges associated with orphanhood, including emotional distress, economic vulnerability, and potential disruptions in education.

Social and Economic Impact: HIV-related orphanhood contributes to the cycle of poverty, affecting children's education, nutrition, and overall well being.

- **Access to Education and Support:**

Educational Disparities: The impact of HIV on families can result in educational disparities for children, particularly when parental illness or death affects their ability to attend school.

Community and Social Support: Building supportive communities and social networks is crucial for women and children affected by HIV. Supportive environments can mitigate the impact of stigma and contribute to improved mental health.

- **Prevention and Support Strategies:**

Prevention Programs for Women: Tailoring prevention programs to address the specific needs of women, including access to female-controlled prevention methods like preexposure prophylaxis (PrEP),

Integrated Health Services: Providing integrated healthcare services that address both HIV and reproductive health needs can improve outcomes for women.

Pediatric Care and Support: Ensuring access to comprehensive pediatric care, including early HIV testing and treatment, for children born to HIV-positive mothers

Supportive Policies: Advocating for policies that address gender inequalities, protect the rights of women and children affected by HIV, and promote access to education and healthcare

In conclusion, addressing the impact of HIV on women and children requires a comprehensive approach that considers biological, social, and economic factors. Efforts should focus on prevention, early diagnosis, access to treatment, and the creation of supportive environments that empower women and children to lead healthy and fulfilling lives in the context of HIV/AIDS.

CHAPTER 8: HIV/AIDS EDUCATION AND AWARENESS PROGRAMS

HIV/AIDS education and awareness programs are essential components of public health initiatives aimed at preventing new infections, dispelling myths, reducing stigma, and promoting overall well being. These programs employ various strategies to reach diverse populations, including schools, communities, and through media channels.

Effective educational strategies

Effective educational strategies are critical in the context of HIV/AIDS to ensure that individuals receive accurate information, are empowered to make informed decisions, and can actively contribute to the prevention of new infections. These strategies encompass various approaches, from formal classroom education to community workshops and online resources.

Here are key elements of effective educational strategies for HIV/AIDS:

- **Comprehensive Sex Education (CSE):**

Inclusion of HIV Content: Comprehensive sex education should include dedicated content on HIV/AIDS, covering topics such as transmission, prevention methods (including condoms and preexposure prophylaxis, PrEP), and the importance of regular testing.

Holistic Approach: CSE should take a holistic approach, addressing not only the biological aspects of HIV but also the social, emotional, and cultural dimensions of sexuality. This includes discussions on healthy relationships, communication skills, and consent.

Age-appropriate Information: Tailoring the information to the age and developmental stage of the audience is crucial. Age-appropriate content ensures that individuals receive information that is relevant to their understanding and experiences.

- **Peer Education Programs**:

Youth Engagement: peer educators, especially within younger age groups, facilitate discussions and share information in a relatable manner. Peers can be effective messengers in conveying messages about HIV prevention.

Interactive Sessions: Peer-led interactive sessions can include group discussions, role playing, and other activities that engage learners and encourage open dialogue about HIV/AIDS.

Empowerment and Skill Building: Empowering individuals with knowledge and skills to make informed decisions about their sexual health This includes teaching effective communication, negotiation skills, and decision-making.

- **Community Workshops and Outreach:**

Targeted Workshops: Conducting workshops within communities that address specific issues related to HIV/AIDS Workshops can cover topics such as stigma, discrimination, and cultural factors influencing HIV risk.

Testing and Counseling Services: Integrating HIV testing and counseling services into community outreach programs to make these services more accessible and reduce the fear associated with testing

Cultural Competency: ensuring that educational materials and workshops are culturally competent, taking into account local customs, languages, and beliefs to make information relatable and acceptable.

- **Online and Technology-Based Education:**

Webinars and Online Courses: Utilizing online platforms to disseminate information to a wider audience Webinars, online courses, and educational videos can provide convenient access to information.

Mobile Apps: Developing mobile applications that offer educational content, resources, and tools for individuals to learn about and manage their sexual health Apps can also provide information on nearby testing centers.

Interactive and Gamified Content: Creating interactive and gamified educational content that engages users and makes learning about HIV/AIDS an enjoyable and memorable experience

- **Culturally Tailored Approaches:**

Understanding Local Contexts: Designing educational materials and strategies that are culturally sensitive and relevant to the specific needs of diverse populations. This includes considering linguistic diversity, cultural norms, and religious beliefs.

Involvement of Community Leaders: Engaging community leaders and influencers in the development and delivery of educational programs to enhance credibility and acceptance within the community

Community Participation: Encouraging active participation of community members in the design and implementation of educational programs to ensure that the content resonates with the local context.

- **Interactive Learning Activities**:

RolePlaying and Simulations: Incorporating roleplaying and simulations in educational sessions to help individuals practice communication and negotiation skills in various situations

Case Studies and Real-Life Examples: Using case studies and real-life examples to illustrate the impact of

HIV/AIDS, challenges faced by individuals, and successful prevention strategies

Question and Answer Sessions: Facilitating open question and answer sessions to address individual concerns and provide clarifications on misconceptions related to HIV/AIDS

- **Evaluation and Feedback Mechanisms:**

Assessment Tools: Incorporating assessment tools to gauge the effectiveness of educational programs This can include pre- and post-assessments to measure changes in knowledge and attitudes.

Feedback Loops: Establishing feedback loops to collect input from participants and stakeholders This feedback can inform improvements in the design and delivery of educational programs.

Continuous Improvement: Being responsive to the evolving needs of the community by continuously evaluating and updating educational materials and approaches.

In conclusion, effective educational strategies for HIV/AIDS involve a combination of comprehensive sex education, peer-led initiatives, community engagement, and innovative technology-based approaches. By considering cultural sensitivities, encouraging active participation, and incorporating interactive learning activities, these strategies contribute to building a well-informed and empowered community in the fight against HIV/AIDS.

Promoting awareness in schools and communities

Promoting awareness of HIV/AIDS in schools and communities is crucial for preventing new infections, challenging stigma, and fostering a supportive environment. Tailoring awareness programs to the specific needs of diverse populations within schools and communities ensures that information is relevant, accessible, and effectively communicated.

Here are key elements of promoting awareness in schools and communities:

- **School-Based Awareness Programs**:

Incorporating HIV Education into Curricula:

Comprehensive Sex Education (CSE): Integrating age-appropriate information about HIV/AIDS into comprehensive sex education curricula to provide students with a foundational understanding of the virus

Health Education: including dedicated units on HIV/AIDS within broader health education programs, covering topics such as transmission, prevention, testing, and the importance of destigmatizing the virus.

Creating Safe Spaces:

Non-discriminatory environment: Fostering a school environment that is free from discrimination based on HIV status or sexual orientation This includes promoting inclusivity and tolerance.

Supportive Counseling Services: Offering counseling services within schools to address the mental health needs of students affected by HIV, whether directly or indirectly.

StudentLed Initiatives:

Peer Education Programs: Implementing peer-led initiatives where students are trained as peer educators to disseminate information about HIV/AIDS among their peers

Youth clubs and organizations: Establishing youth clubs or organizations that focus on promoting awareness, challenging stigma, and organizing events within the school community

- **Community Engagement and Outreach:**

Workshops and Events:
Community Workshops: Conducting workshops within communities to provide information about HIV transmission, prevention methods, and the importance of testing. These workshops can be tailored to specific community needs.

Health Fairs: Organizing health fairs that include HIV testing services, educational booths, and interactive activities to engage community members in discussions about HIV/AIDS.

Faith-Based Initiatives:
Collaboration with Religious Leaders: Collaborating with religious leaders and organizations to incorporate HIV education into religious teachings and community activities

Community Dialogues: Facilitating community dialogues that involve religious leaders, community members, and healthcare professionals to address cultural and religious perspectives on HIV/AIDS.

Community-Based Organizations:
Collaboration with NGOs: Partnering with nongovernmental organizations (NGOs) and community-based organizations that specialize in HIV/AIDS awareness and support services.

Community Health Workers: Engaging community health workers to conduct door-to-door outreach, provide information, and encourage individuals to get tested for HIV.

- **Media and Communication Strategies:**

Public Service Announcements (PSAs):
Television and Radio PSAs: Creating short and impactful public service announcements that communicate key messages about HIV prevention, testing, and destigmatization.

Print media: publishing informative articles, infographics, and editorials in local newspapers and magazines to reach a broader audience.

Social Media Campaigns:

Hashtag Campaigns: Launching social media campaigns with relevant hashtags to promote awareness, share information, and encourage open discussions about HIV/AIDS.

Influencer Partnerships: Collaborating with social media influencers and local celebrities to amplify awareness messages and reach diverse audiences.

Interactive Platforms:

Online Webinars and Q&A Sessions: Conducting online webinars and question-and-answer sessions to engage the community in discussions about HIV/AIDS.

Interactive Websites and Apps: Developing interactive websites and mobile applications that provide educational content, resources, and tools for individuals to learn more about HIV/AIDS.

- **Legal Protections and Anti-Discrimination Efforts**:

Incorporating legal information: Including information on legal protections against HIV-related discrimination and stigma in awareness campaigns to empower individuals and educate them about their rights.

Advocacy Efforts: Engaging in advocacy efforts to promote and strengthen legal protections for individuals living with HIV, ensuring they are not unfairly treated in schools or communities.

Promoting Inclusivity: Encouraging schools and communities to adopt policies that promote inclusivity, protect against discrimination, and provide support for those affected by HIV/AIDS.

- **Evaluation and Feedback Mechanisms:**

Assessment Tools: Incorporating assessment tools to gauge the effectiveness of awareness programs This may involve pre- and post-assessments to measure changes in knowledge and attitudes.

Community Feedback Sessions: Hosting feedback sessions within schools and communities to collect input from participants. This feedback can inform improvements in the design and delivery of awareness programs.

Continuous Improvement: Regularly evaluating and updating awareness materials and approaches based on the feedback received and the evolving needs of the community.

In conclusion, promoting awareness of HIV/AIDS in schools and communities requires a multifaceted approach that includes comprehensive education, community engagement, media campaigns, legal protections, and ongoing evaluation. By addressing the unique needs of different populations and fostering an environment of openness and support, these initiatives contribute to the broader goal of preventing new infections and building informed and empowered communities.

The role of media and social campaigns

The role of media and social campaigns is pivotal in the realm of HIV/AIDS awareness and prevention. These campaigns leverage various communication channels to disseminate accurate information, challenge stigma, promote testing, and encourage positive behavioral changes. Here's an exploration of the key aspects of the role of media and social campaigns in the context of HIV/AIDS:

- **Public Service Announcements (PSAs):**

Television and Radio PSAs: Short and impactful messages broadcast on television and radio platforms are essential for reaching a broad audience. PSAs can convey critical information about HIV transmission, prevention methods, and the importance of testing.

Message Clarity and Simplicity: PSAs focus on delivering clear and simple messages to ensure easy comprehension and retention by the audience. Visual and auditory elements are carefully crafted for maximum impact.

- **Print and Online Media:**

Printed Materials: Informative articles, brochures, posters, and pamphlets distributed in healthcare settings, schools, and public spaces contribute to disseminating accurate information about HIV/AIDS.

Online Platforms and Websites: Developing informative websites, online articles, and blogs helps reach audiences who prefer digital sources. Interactive features and multimedia content enhance engagement.

Infographics and Visual Aids: Visual aids, including infographics and charts, play a crucial role in conveying complex information in a visually appealing and easily digestible format.

- **Social Media Campaign**s:

Hashtag Campaigns: Launching campaigns with relevant hashtags on platforms like Twitter, Instagram, and TikTok facilitates the creation of a digital conversation around HIV/AIDS. It encourages users to share information, personal stories, and resources.

Influencer Partnerships: Collaborating with social media influencers and celebrities helps amplify the reach of awareness messages. Influencers can use their platforms to share accurate information, reduce stigma, and encourage testing.

Interactive Content: Creating quizzes, polls, and interactive content on social media platforms engages the audience actively and promotes knowledge retention.

- **Documentaries and Films:**

Narrative Storytelling: Documentaries and films provide a platform for narrative storytelling, allowing individuals to share their experiences with HIV/AIDS. This humanizes the impact of the virus, fostering empathy and understanding.

Educational Films: Producing educational films that are both informative and emotionally resonant contributes to destigmatizing HIV/AIDS and challenging misconceptions.

- **Community Engagement:**

Community Dialogues: Media campaigns can facilitate community dialogues, bringing together diverse voices to discuss HIV/AIDS openly. These discussions can address cultural nuances, dispel myths, and promote community-wide understanding.

Coverage of LocalInitiatives:: Media outlets can cover and highlight local initiatives, events, and success stories related to HIV/AIDS awareness within communities. This helps build a sense of pride and shared responsibility.

- **Interactive Workshops and Events:**

Media-Supported Events: Hosting events in collaboration with media outlets can enhance the visibility and impact of workshops and awareness campaigns. Live streaming and coverage can extend the reach to a wider audience.

Celebrity Endorsements and Participation: Involving celebrities and public figures in workshops and events not only attracts attention but also brings credibility to the cause. Their participation can encourage more individuals to engage with the campaign.

- **Multilingual and Culturally Sensitive Content:**

Language Diversity: Recognizing the diversity of languages spoken within a community and creating content in multiple languages ensures inclusivity and broadens the reach of campaigns.

Cultural Competency: Adapting content to be culturally sensitive is crucial. Understanding cultural norms, beliefs, and practices helps in crafting messages that resonate positively with the target audience.

- **Evaluation and Impact Assessment:**

Monitoring Reach and Engagement: Tracking the reach and engagement of media and social campaigns provides insights into their effectiveness. Metrics such as views, shares, and comments help assess impact.

Assessment of Knowledge Gain: Implementing pre- and post-campaign surveys to measure changes in knowledge, attitudes, and behaviors helps in understanding the campaign's influence.

Feedback Mechanisms: Establishing feedback mechanisms, such as online surveys and community forums, allows participants to share their thoughts, suggestions, and concerns, contributing to ongoing improvements.

In conclusion, the role of media and social campaigns in raising HIV/AIDS awareness is multifaceted. These campaigns have the power to inform, inspire, and mobilize communities toward positive behavioral changes. By leveraging various communication channels and adopting culturally sensitive approaches, media and social campaigns play a crucial role in the global effort to combat HIV/AIDS.

CHAPTER 9: GLOBAL EFFORTS AND INITIATIVES

Global efforts and initiatives in the fight against HIV/AIDS involve the collaboration of international organizations, governments, nonprofits, healthcare providers, and communities. These efforts aim to reduce new infections, improve access to treatment and care, and address the social and economic impact of the HIV/AIDS pandemic.

Overview of international organizations fighting HIV/AIDS

International organizations play a crucial role in the global fight against HIV/AIDS, providing coordination, funding, technical assistance, and advocacy to address the multifaceted challenges posed by the epidemic.

Here's an overview of key international organizations dedicated to combating HIV/AIDS:

1. **Joint United Nations Programme on HIV/AIDS (UNAIDS):**

Mandate: UNAIDS was established in 1996 and is the main advocate for global action against HIV/AIDS. It brings together 11 UN agencies, including WHO, UNICEF, and UNDP, to coordinate international efforts.

Roles and Responsibilities: UNAIDS provides strategic leadership, advocates for political commitment, mobilizes resources, and supports countries in their response to HIV/AIDS. It works towards global goals such as the 909090 targets (90% of people living with HIV knowing their status, 90% of diagnosed individuals on treatment, and 90% of those on treatment having suppressed viral loads).

2. World Health Organization (WHO):

Mandate: WHO is the global health agency of the United Nations. It provides leadership on global health matters, shaping the health research agenda, setting norms and standards, and providing technical support to countries.

Roles and Responsibilities: WHO plays a central role in providing technical guidance on HIV prevention, treatment, and care. It sets global norms, supports capacity building, and monitors progress towards global targets.

3. Global Fund to Fight AIDS, Tuberculosis, and Malaria:

Mandate: The Global Fund is a financing organization established in 2002 to accelerate the end of the three epidemics—HIV/AIDS, tuberculosis, and malaria.

Roles and Responsibilities: The Global Fund provides funding to countries for programs that aim to prevent and treat HIV/AIDS. It operates through a partnership model, working with governments, civil society, and the private sector.

4. PEPFAR (President's Emergency Plan for AIDS Relief):

Mandate: PEPFAR is a United States government initiative launched in 2003 to combat the global HIV/AIDS epidemic.

Roles and responsibilities: PEPFAR provides funding and technical assistance to countries heavily affected by HIV/AIDS. It supports a range of activities, including prevention, testing, treatment, and care. PEPFAR focuses on implementing evidence-based interventions to achieve epidemic control.

5. UNITAID:

Mandate: UNITAID was established in 2006 to increase access to treatment for HIV/AIDS, tuberculosis, and malaria by leveraging innovative financing mechanisms.

Roles and Responsibilities: UNITAID works to accelerate the development and scaleup of innovative health solutions, including new drugs, diagnostics, and prevention tools. It operates at the intersection of public health, intellectual property, and market dynamics.

6. Global HIV Vaccine Enterprise:

Mandate: The Global HIV Vaccine Enterprise is an alliance of researchers, funders, and advocates dedicated to accelerating the development of a preventive HIV vaccine.

Roles and Responsibilities: The enterprise coordinates global efforts to overcome scientific, technical, and social challenges in HIV vaccine development. It facilitates collaboration and information sharing among stakeholders.

7. UNICEF (United Nations International Children's Emergency Fund):

Mandate: UNICEF is a UN agency focused on the wellbeing of children and mothers.

Roles and Responsibilities: UNICEF plays a critical role in supporting programs for the prevention of mother-to-child transmission (PMTCT) of HIV. It works to ensure that children affected by HIV/AIDS have access to essential services, including education and healthcare.

8. UNDP (United Nations Development Programme):

Mandate: UNDP works to eradicate poverty, reduce inequalities, and build resilience to crises.

Roles and Responsibilities: UNDP supports countries in integrating HIV/AIDS responses into broader development strategies. It focuses on addressing social and economic determinants of HIV, promoting human rights, and strengthening community engagement.

These international organizations collaborate with governments, civil society, and the private sector to implement evidence-based interventions, mobilize resources, and advocate for policies that support the global response to HIV/AIDS. Through their collective efforts, progress has been made, but challenges remain in achieving the goal of ending the AIDS epidemic by 2030.

Success stories and challenges in different regions

Success stories and challenges in the global fight against HIV/AIDS vary across regions due to diverse social, economic, and cultural contexts. While there have been notable achievements, persistent challenges underscore the need for continued efforts. Here's an overview of success stories and challenges in different regions:

- **SubSaharan Africa:**

Success Stories:

Increased Access to Treatment: SubSaharan Africa has made significant strides in expanding access to antiretroviral therapy (ART), resulting in improved health outcomes for people living with HIV.

Prevention of Mother-to-Child Transmission (PMTCT): Successes in PMTCT programs have led to a reduction in the number of children born with HIV.

Community-led initiatives: community-based organizations and initiatives have played a vital role in raising awareness, promoting testing, and providing support to those affected.

Challenges:

High Prevalence Rates: The region bears a disproportionate burden of the global HIV/AIDS epidemic, with high prevalence rates in many countries.

Stigma and Discrimination: Stigma remains a significant barrier to testing and treatment, leading to late diagnosis and increased transmission.

Resource Constraints: Some countries face challenges in mobilizing adequate resources for sustained prevention and treatment efforts.

- **Asia and the Pacific:**

Success Stories:

Scaling Up Treatment: Several countries in the region have successfully scaled up HIV treatment programs, **reaching a greater number of individuals in need.**

Innovative Approaches: Implementation of innovative strategies, such as harm reduction programs for key populations, has shown positive results.

Increased Testing Rates: Efforts to promote HIV testing have contributed to a better understanding of the epidemic's scope.

Challenges:

Stigma and Discrimination: Stigma remains a significant barrier to testing and treatment adherence, particularly for key populations.

Access to Treatment in Remote Areas: Limited access to healthcare services in remote areas poses challenges to timely diagnosis and treatment.

Emerging Challenges among Youth: An emerging concern is the rising number of new infections among young people, highlighting the need for targeted prevention efforts.

- **Latin America and the Caribbean:**

Success Stories:

Reduction in New Infections: Some countries have experienced a decline in new HIV infections, attributed to successful prevention programs.

Increased Testing and Treatment: Efforts to promote testing and expand access to treatment have contributed to improved outcomes.

Community-Led Initiatives: Communitybased organizations have been instrumental in reaching key populations and advocating for their rights.

Challenges:

Inequalities and Disparities: Inequalities in access to healthcare and prevention services persist, particularly among marginalized populations.

Stigma and Discrimination: Stigma remains a challenge, affecting testing rates and the overall quality of life for people living with HIV.

Sustainable Funding: Securing sustainable funding for HIV programs and ensuring their integration into broader health systems pose ongoing challenges.

- **Eastern Europe and Central Asia:**

Success Stories:

Improved Testing and Surveillance: Some countries have enhanced HIV testing and surveillance, leading to a better understanding of the epidemic.

Community Engagement: The increasing involvement of communities in advocacy and service delivery has shown positive results.

Policy Reforms: Several countries have made policy changes to support harm reduction approaches for people who inject drugs.

Challenges:

Increasing New Infections: The region has seen an increase in new HIV infections, particularly among key populations.

Stigma and Criminalization: Stigma, discrimination, and the criminalization of certain behaviors hinder prevention efforts and access to services.

Limited Resources: Resource constraints and competing health priorities pose challenges to sustaining effective HIV programs.

These regional examples highlight the importance of tailoring interventions to local contexts, addressing social determinants, and fostering collaborative efforts between governments, civil society, and international partners. While progress has been made, the persistence of challenges underscores the ongoing need for comprehensive and sustained efforts to achieve the goal of ending the AIDS epidemic.

The importance of collaboration on a global scale

Collaboration on a global scale is paramount to addressing complex challenges such as HIV/AIDS. The interconnected nature of the epidemic, with its social, economic, and public health dimensions, necessitates concerted efforts from governments, international organizations, NGOs, healthcare professionals, researchers, and affected communities.

Here's an exploration of the importance of global collaboration in the fight against HIV/AIDS:

- **Pooling Resources and Expertise:**

Financial Resources: Global collaboration enables the pooling of financial resources from various countries and organizations. This collective funding helps support comprehensive prevention, treatment, and care programs.

Technical Expertise: Different regions and organizations bring unique technical expertise. Collaboration allows for the sharing of knowledge, best practices, and innovations, contributing to more effective strategies.

- **Ensuring Universal Access to Treatment and Care:**

Equitable Distribution of Resources: Global collaboration helps address disparities in resource distribution, ensuring that even resource-constrained regions have access to essential medications, diagnostics, and healthcare infrastructure.

Preventing Drug Stockouts: Cooperation on a global scale helps prevent interruptions in the supply chain of antiretroviral drugs, ensuring that individuals receive consistent and uninterrupted treatment.

- **Research and Innovation:**

Accelerating Research: Global collaboration accelerates the pace of research and development. By bringing together researchers and institutions worldwide, breakthroughs in prevention methods, treatment modalities, and potential vaccines are more likely.

Learning from Diverse Experiences: Different regions face unique challenges. Collaboration allows researchers and policymakers to learn from diverse experiences and adapt interventions to specific contexts.

- **Advocacy and Political Will:**

Amplifying Voices: Collaborative efforts amplify the voices of those affected by HIV/AIDS. Advocacy on a global scale can draw attention to the importance of sustained political will, resulting in increased commitment from governments and policymakers.

Addressing Social Determinants: HIV/AIDS is intricately linked to social determinants such as poverty, gender inequality, and discrimination. Global collaboration enables advocacy for broader social and economic changes that address these determinants.

- **Prevention Strategies and Education:**

Scaling Up Prevention Programs: Collaborative initiatives enable the scaling up of evidence-based prevention programs. This includes educational campaigns, condom distribution, and harm reduction strategies.

Reaching Vulnerable Populations: Global collaboration is crucial in reaching key populations, such as sex workers, men who have sex with men, and people who inject drugs. These groups often face increased vulnerability to HIV/AIDS due to stigma, discrimination, and legal barriers.

- **Monitoring and Evaluation:**

Global Metrics and Targets: Collaboration allows for the establishment of global metrics and targets, such as the 90 90 90 goals set by UNAIDS. These goals provide a framework for monitoring progress and identifying areas that need additional attention.

Data Sharing: Collaborative efforts in data collection and sharing contribute to a more comprehensive understanding of the epidemic's dynamics. This data informs decision-making and resource allocation.

- **Capacity Building and Training:**

Building Local Capacities: Global collaboration supports capacity building in affected regions. This includes training healthcare professionals, community workers, and researchers to strengthen local responses to HIV/AIDS.

Knowledge Transfer: Collaboration facilitates the transfer of knowledge and skills between regions, ensuring that best practices are disseminated and implemented in diverse settings.

- **Addressing Human Rights and Stigma:**

International Advocacy: Collaborative efforts on a global scale contribute to international advocacy for human rights and the reduction of stigma. This includes efforts to decriminalize certain behaviors associated with HIV/AIDS.

Legal Protections: Global collaboration can influence the development and strengthening of legal protections for individuals living with HIV, promoting nondiscrimination and the protection of their rights.

- **Preparing for Emerging Challenges**:

Anticipating and Responding to Emerging Threats: Global collaboration prepares the world to respond to emerging challenges, such as new strains of the virus, potential drug resistance, and unforeseen public health crises.

Coordination in Pandemics: Lessons learned from the global response to HIV/AIDS contribute to effective coordination in addressing other pandemics, such as the response to COVID-19.

In conclusion, the importance of collaboration on a global scale in the fight against HIV/AIDS cannot be overstated. It is a collective endeavor that draws on the strengths of diverse stakeholders to tackle the multifaceted challenges posed by the epidemic. Through collaborative efforts, progress is made toward the goal of ending the AIDS epidemic, and the lessons learned contribute to broader global health initiatives and responses.

CHAPTER 10: LIVING WITH HIV/AIDS

Living with HIV/AIDS presents unique challenges, but with advancements in medical care and a supportive environment, individuals with HIV can lead healthy and fulfilling lives.

Coping with an HIV diagnosis

Coping with an HIV diagnosis is a significant and often challenging life event. The emotional impact, fear of the unknown, and concerns about the future can be overwhelming. However, with the right support, resources, and coping strategies, individuals can navigate this journey and lead healthy, fulfilling lives.

Here are some key aspects of coping with an HIV diagnosis:

- **Emotional Impact:**

Initial Reactions: Receiving an HIV diagnosis can trigger a range of emotions, including shock, fear, sadness, anger, and anxiety. It's essential to acknowledge and accept these emotions as a natural response to a life-changing event.

Stigma and Shame: Stigma associated with HIV/AIDS can contribute to feelings of shame and isolation. Understanding that HIV is a medical condition and not a moral judgment is crucial for coping with societal perceptions.

Grief and Loss: Individuals may experience a sense of loss, including the loss of perceived health, future plans, and a sense of control. Coping involves allowing oneself to grieve while also seeking support to navigate these emotions.

- **Seeking Professional Support**:

Counseling and Therapy: Mental health professionals, such as psychologists or counselors, can provide a safe space to discuss emotions, fears, and concerns. Therapy can help individuals develop coping strategies and resilience.

Support Groups: Joining HIV support groups allows individuals to connect with others who share similar experiences. Sharing stories, advice, and coping mechanisms in a supportive environment can be immensely beneficial.

Peer Counseling: Engaging with peer counselors who are also living with HIV can provide a unique and relatable source of support. Peer counseling fosters a sense of community and understanding.

- **Educational Resources**:

Understanding HIV: Learning about HIV, its transmission, treatment options, and how to maintain a healthy lifestyle is empowering. Accurate information dispels myths and helps individuals make informed decisions about their health.

Treatment Options: Knowing about available treatment options, including antiretroviral therapy (ART), and understanding the importance of adherence helps individuals take an active role in managing their health.

- **Building a Support Network**:

Family and Friends: Open communication with family and friends is crucial. Sharing one's diagnosis can strengthen relationships and create a supportive network.

Partner Support: If applicable, involving a partner in the journey can enhance emotional support and facilitate shared decision-making, including discussions about safe practices.

Social Connections: Maintaining social connections with friends and community helps combat isolation. It's essential to foster relationships that provide encouragement and understanding.

- **Self-care strategies**:

Healthy Lifestyle Choices: Adopting a healthy lifestyle, including regular exercise, a balanced diet, and adequate sleep, contributes to overall wellbeing. These factors can also positively impact the immune system.

Stress Management: Learning and practicing stress management techniques, such as mindfulness, meditation, or yoga, can help alleviate the emotional burden associated with an HIV diagnosis.

Balancing Work and Health: Finding a balance between work or other responsibilities and health management is crucial. This may involve adjustments to work schedules or seeking support from employers.

- **Legal and advocacy support:**

Understanding Rights: Knowing one's legal rights, including protections against discrimination, is important. Advocacy organizations often provide information and support in navigating legal matters.

Participation in Advocacy: Some individuals find empowerment and purpose in participating in advocacy efforts to reduce HIV stigma, raise awareness, and promote access to healthcare.

Coping with an HIV diagnosis is a personal and ongoing process. It involves adapting to new realities, seeking support, and making informed choices about healthcare. As medical advancements continue, the outlook for individuals living with HIV has improved significantly, emphasizing the importance of early diagnosis, access to treatment, and holistic support.

Support networks and resources

Support networks and resources play a crucial role in the lives of individuals living with HIV. These networks provide emotional support, facilitate access to information, and contribute to an overall sense of community.

Here's an exploration of the various support networks and resources available for individuals living with HIV:

- **Healthcare Providers and Services:**

Infectious Disease Specialists: Establishing a relationship with infectious disease specialists and other healthcare providers is fundamental. Regular medical checkups, adherence to treatment plans, and open communication contribute to overall health.

HIV Clinics and Treatment Centers: Specialized clinics and treatment centers often provide comprehensive care for individuals living with HIV. These facilities may offer a range of services, including counseling, support groups, and access to the latest treatments.

- **Community-Based Organizations and Support Groups:**

Local NGOs and Community Centers: Nonprofit organizations and community centers often provide a range of services, including counseling, support groups, and educational programs. These organizations may address the broader needs of individuals living with HIV, such as housing, legal support, and nutrition assistance.

Support Groups for People Living with HIV (PLHIV): Joining support groups specifically for individuals living with HIV offers a space to share experiences, discuss common challenges, and receive emotional support. These groups may be facilitated by healthcare professionals or community leaders.

- **Online Communities and Forums:**

Virtual Support Networks: Online communities and forums provide a platform for individuals living with HIV to connect with others globally. These platforms allow for anonymous discussions, information sharing, and the opportunity to seek advice from peers.

Social Media Groups: Various social media platforms host groups and pages dedicated to individuals living with HIV. These spaces foster a sense of community and enable people to share their stories and insights.

- **Mental Health Professionals:**

Psychologists and Counselors: Mental health professionals specializing in HIV/AIDS can offer support in coping with the emotional and psychological aspects of living with the virus. Counseling sessions can address concerns such as stigma, depression, and anxiety.

Psychiatric Support: For individuals dealing with more severe mental health issues, psychiatric support may be necessary. Professionals can provide a range of interventions, including medication management and therapeutic approaches.

- **Legal Support and Advocacy Organizations:**

Legal Protections: Organizations specializing in legal support can provide information on legal protections against discrimination based on HIV status. They may also offer assistance in cases where individuals face discrimination or legal challenges.

Advocacy Groups: Advocacy organizations work to reduce stigma, improve access to healthcare, and promote the rights of individuals living with HIV. These groups often engage in policy advocacy, community education, and awareness campaigns.

- **Family and Friends**:

Personal Support Network: Family and friends can offer a crucial personal support network. Open communication, understanding, and encouragement from loved ones contribute to emotional wellbeing.

Education for Loved Ones: Providing educational resources to family and friends helps them better understand HIV/AIDS, reduces stigma, and fosters a supportive environment.

- **National and International Helplines:**

Hotlines and Helplines: National and international helplines provide immediate support and information. These services are often staffed by trained professionals who can answer questions, offer guidance, and provide crisis intervention.

Crisis Text Lines: Text-based support services are available in some regions, allowing individuals to reach out for assistance via text messages.

- **Religious and Faith-Based Support:**

Faith Communities: Some individuals find support within their religious or faith communities. Clergy, pastoral counselors, or faith leaders may offer spiritual guidance and emotional support.

Religious Support Groups: Some faith-based organizations have support groups specifically for individuals living with HIV, addressing both spiritual and practical aspects of their lives.

Access to these support networks and resources is essential for the holistic wellbeing of individuals living with HIV. These networks not only provide practical assistance but also contribute to reducing stigma, fostering resilience, and empowering individuals to lead healthy and fulfilling lives.

Inspiring stories of individuals living well with HIV

Inspiring stories of individuals living well with HIV showcase resilience, strength, and the transformative power of medical advancements and social support. These narratives challenge stereotypes, reduce stigma, and provide hope for others facing a similar diagnosis.
 Here are a few examples of inspiring stories:

1. Magic Johnson:

Background: Perhaps one of the best-known stories, Earvin "Magic" Johnson, the legendary basketball player, publicly disclosed his HIV positive status in 1991, shocking the world.

Living Well with HIV: Magic Johnson's Story is a testament to the advances in HIV treatment. Through a combination of early detection, access to quality healthcare, and adherence to antiretroviral therapy (ART), he has not only survived but thrived.

Advocacy: Magic Johnson became a prominent advocate for HIV awareness and prevention. His story highlights the importance of using one's platform to educate and reduce stigma.

2. Hydeia Broadbent:

Background: Diagnosed with HIV at birth in 1984, Hydeia Broadbent has lived her entire life with the virus.

Advocacy and Education: Despite facing numerous challenges, Hydeia has become a powerful HIV advocate and educator. She has been a vocal spokesperson, emphasizing the importance of testing, early treatment, and breaking down misconceptions about HIV.

Living Positively: Hydeia's story illustrates that with proper care, individuals living with HIV from a young age can lead positive and impactful lives.

3. Rae Lewis Thornton:

Background: Diagnosed with HIV in 1986, Rae Lewis Thornton has been living with the virus for over three decades.

Public Speaker and Activist: Rae is a public speaker, author, and HIV/AIDS activist. She uses her platform to challenge stereotypes and speak about her journey with

HIV, including the complexities of living with a chronic illness.

Educating and Empowering Others: Rae's story emphasizes the importance of education, destigmatization, and the power of individuals to live full lives despite a chronic health condition.

4. Andrew Pulsipher:

Background: Born with HIV in 1981, Andrew Pulsipher has never known life without the virus.

Healthy Family and Advocacy: Andrew is a father of three HIV-negative children and is living proof that with proper medical care and precautions, the risk of mother-to-child transmission can be greatly minimized.

Breaking Stigmas: Andrew's story challenges common misconceptions about HIV transmission within families and highlights the potential for individuals with HIV to lead fulfilling family lives.

5. Maria Mejia:

Background: Maria Mejia, diagnosed with HIV in 1991, has faced stigma and discrimination throughout her life.

Advocacy for Women and Latinx Community: Maria has become a powerful advocate for women living with HIV and the Latinx community. She speaks openly about her experiences to reduce stigma, raise awareness, and promote empowerment.

Social Media Influence: Maria uses social media platforms to share her journey and connect with others. Her story illustrates the impact of personal narratives on fostering understanding and support.

6. Gus Cairns:

Background: Gus Cairns, a prominent HIV journalist, was diagnosed in 1993.

Advocacy through Journalism: Gus has used his career to advocate for HIV awareness and challenge misconceptions. His journalistic work has contributed to reducing stigma and providing accurate information.

Living Positively in Later Years: Gus Cairns' story demonstrates that individuals diagnosed with HIV in the early years of the epidemic can live into later life with proper care and treatment.

These stories reflect the diversity of experiences within the HIV community and the impact of positive living, access to healthcare, and advocacy. They show that living well with HIV is not only possible but can also be accompanied by personal growth, resilience, and the ability to make a positive impact on others.

CHAPTER 11: FUTURE DIRECTIONS IN HIV PREVENTION AND RESEARCH

Future directions in HIV prevention and research are characterized by ongoing efforts to enhance current prevention methods, explore new breakthroughs, and pursue the ultimate goal of developing a safe and effective HIV vaccine.

Current Research and Breakthroughs

Long-Acting Antiretrovirals (ARVs): Research is focusing on developing long-acting formulations of antiretroviral drugs to reduce the frequency of medication administration. Injectable ARVs that provide protection for several weeks or months are being investigated, potentially improving adherence and effectiveness.

Treatment as Prevention (TasP): The concept of using HIV treatment as a form of prevention has gained prominence. Early initiation of antiretroviral therapy not only benefits the individual but also significantly reduces the risk of transmitting the virus to others.

Pre-Exposure Prophylaxis (PrEP) Innovations: While oral PrEP has proven highly effective, researchers are exploring alternative delivery methods, such as injectable PrEP, implantable devices, and on-demand PrEP. These innovations aim to address issues related to adherence and accessibility.

Microbicides and Topical Prevention: Research continues on the development of microbicides—topical substances that can be applied to the genital or rectal mucosa to prevent HIV transmission. This approach provides an additional tool for individuals who may face challenges with other prevention methods.

Gene Editing Technologies: Emerging technologies like CRISPRCas9 are being explored for potential use in editing the genetic material of cells susceptible to HIV infection. While this area is in the early stages of research, it holds promise for developing novel prevention strategies.

Promising Prevention Methods on the Horizon

Broadly Neutralizing Antibodies (bNAbs): Investigational monoclonal antibodies with the ability to neutralize a broad range of HIV strains are being studied. These antibodies could be used for both treatment and prevention, offering an additional layer of protection.

Nanoparticle Vaccines: Nanoparticle-based vaccines are being developed to mimic the structure of the HIV virus, prompting a targeted immune response. These vaccine candidates aim to induce broadly neutralizing antibodies and elicit a more effective immune defense.

Passive Immunization Strategies: Passive immunization involves providing individuals with preformed antibodies, offering immediate protection against HIV. This approach is being explored as both a preventive measure and a potential treatment strategy.

The Quest for an HIV Vaccine

Ongoing Vaccine Trials: Several HIV vaccine candidates are currently undergoing clinical trials. These trials aim to evaluate the safety, immunogenicity, and efficacy of potential vaccines in diverse populations.

Mosaic Vaccines: Mosaic vaccines are designed to elicit immune responses against a variety of HIV strains. They incorporate components from multiple HIV subtypes, potentially providing broader protection. Clinical trials for mosaic vaccines are underway.

RNA Vaccine Technology: RNA vaccine platforms, similar to those used in the development of COVID-19 vaccines, are being explored for HIV. This technology has the potential for rapid development and may contribute to the ongoing quest for an effective HIV vaccine.

Collaborative Global Efforts: Collaborative efforts, involving organizations like the Global HIV Vaccine Enterprise, aim to coordinate and accelerate research in the quest for an HIV vaccine. These efforts prioritize collaboration between researchers, funders, and affected communities.

While significant progress has been made in HIV prevention and research, challenges remain. These challenges include the complexity of the virus, the need for effective and scalable prevention methods, and the importance of addressing social determinants of HIV transmission. Continued investment, international collaboration, and a multifaceted approach are critical to achieving the goal of ending the HIV/AIDS epidemic.

CHAPTER 12: TAKING ACTION: HOW YOU CAN HELP

Taking action to support the fight against HIV/AIDS involves a range of activities, from volunteering and fundraising to advocating for policy change. Individuals can contribute in various ways to make a positive impact on the lives of those affected by HIV/AIDS.

Volunteering opportunities

Volunteering opportunities in the realm of HIV/AIDS are diverse and provide individuals with a chance to make a meaningful impact on the lives of those affected by the virus. Here are various volunteering opportunities in the field of HIV/AIDS:

- **Local HIV/AIDS Service Organizations:**

Services Provided: Many local organizations focus specifically on HIV/AIDS services. They may offer counseling, testing, support groups, and educational programs.

Volunteer Roles: Volunteers can assist with organizing and promoting events, providing support to individuals living with HIV, participating in outreach programs, and contributing to administrative tasks.

- **HIV Testing and Counseling Centers:**

Services Provided: Testing centers play a crucial role in prevention efforts. They provide HIV testing, counseling, and education to individuals.

Volunteer Roles: Volunteers can help organize and run testing events, provide information about HIV prevention, and offer support to individuals undergoing testing.

- **Health Clinics and Hospitals:**

Services Provided: Hospitals and health clinics often have dedicated programs for HIV/AIDS care. They may offer treatment, counseling, and support services.

Volunteer Roles: Volunteers can assist with patient support, administrative tasks, organizing awareness campaigns, and providing information to patients and their families.

- **Educational Programs in Schools:**

Services Provided: Educational programs in schools aim to raise awareness about HIV/AIDS, promote prevention, and reduce stigma.

Volunteer Roles: Volunteers can participate in or lead educational workshops, discussions, and presentations. They may also assist in organizing school-based events focused on HIV/AIDS awareness.

- **Global Health Initiatives:**

Services Provided: International organizations and NGOs often run global health initiatives addressing HIV/AIDS in different regions.

Volunteer Roles: Opportunities may include working on projects related to HIV prevention, treatment, and support. Volunteers may contribute to community outreach, educational programs, and healthcare delivery in various parts of the world.

- **Community-Based Support Groups:**

Services Provided: Support groups bring together individuals living with HIV for mutual support, information sharing, and community building.

Volunteer Roles: Volunteers can facilitate support group sessions, organize social events, provide transportation assistance, and offer one-on-one support to those in need.

- **Crisis Helplines and Hotlines:**

Services Provided: Helplines and hotlines offer immediate support, information, and counseling to individuals facing crises related to HIV/AIDS.

Volunteer Roles: Volunteers can staff helplines, providing a listening ear, offering information, and directing callers to appropriate resources. Training in crisis intervention may be required.

- **Event Planning and Fundraising:**

Services Provided: Events and fundraising initiatives are vital for generating funds to support HIV/AIDS programs and services.

Volunteer Roles: Individuals can contribute by helping plan and organize fundraising events, participating in outreach to secure sponsorships, and assisting with logistics during events.

- **Research and Advocacy Organizations:**

Services Provided: Research and advocacy organizations focus on advancing knowledge, influencing policy, and promoting the rights of individuals affected by HIV/AIDS.

Volunteer Roles: Volunteers may assist with data collection, participate in advocacy campaigns, contribute to research initiatives, and support outreach efforts to raise awareness.

- **Online and Virtual Opportunities:**

Services Provided: In the digital age, there are virtual volunteering opportunities that include tasks such as online counseling, content creation, social media management, and virtual support group facilitation.

Volunteer Roles: Individuals with skills in web development, graphic design, social media, or online communication can contribute their expertise to support virtual initiatives.

Before volunteering, it's important to connect with the respective organizations, understand their needs, and undergo any necessary training. Additionally, individuals should be aware of the cultural sensitivity required when working with diverse communities affected by HIV/AIDS. Volunteering is a powerful way to contribute to the fight against HIV/AIDS, and it provides a unique opportunity for personal growth and community impact.

Fundraising and charitable organizations

Fundraising and charitable organizations play a crucial role in supporting HIV/AIDS-related initiatives, including research, prevention programs, treatment access, and support services for individuals and communities affected by the virus. Engaging in fundraising efforts or supporting charitable organizations contributes to the resources needed to address the multifaceted challenges posed by HIV/AIDS.

Fundraising Initiatives:

- **Events and Campaigns:**

Walks, Runs, and **Marathons:** Organizing or participating in events like charity walks or runs dedicated to HIV/AIDS fundraising is a popular and effective method.

Benefit Concerts and Performances: Hosting musical or artistic events where the proceeds go towards HIV/AIDS causes can attract community support.

Online Crowdfunding Campaigns: Platforms like GoFundMe or Kickstarter offer opportunities for individuals to create campaigns for specific HIV/AIDS-related projects.

- **Corporate Partnerships:**

Sponsorship and Donations: Encouraging businesses to sponsor events, make donations, or establish ongoing partnerships with HIV/AIDS charities can provide substantial financial support.

Employee Engagement Programs: Companies can encourage employee participation in fundraising events or establish workplace giving programs.

- **Community Outreach:**

Local Community Events: Engaging with the community through small-scale events, such as bake sales or neighborhood fundraisers, helps raise awareness and funds.

Collaborations with Local Businesses: Partnering with local businesses for fundraising initiatives, where a portion of sales goes to HIV/AIDS causes, can be mutually beneficial.

Charitable Organizations:

- **Global and National Organizations:**

amfAR (The Foundation for AIDS Research): Dedicated to supporting HIV/AIDS research, prevention, and treatment globally

UNAIDS: The joint United Nations program on HIV/AIDS focuses on coordinating international efforts to combat the epidemic.

- **Community-Based Organizations:**

AIDS Service Organizations (ASOs): Local ASOs provide services such as counseling, testing, and support to individuals living with HIV. Examples include GMHC (Gay Men's Health Crisis) in the U.S.

HIV Clinics and Hospitals: Hospitals and clinics often have affiliated foundations that raise funds for HIV/AIDS-related programs.

- **Research and Advocacy Groups:**

AVAC (Global Advocacy for HIV Prevention): Focuses on accelerating the ethical development and global delivery of HIV prevention options.

TAG (Treatment Action Group):advocates for improved treatment access and accelerated research to find a cure for HIV/AIDS.

- **Children and Family-Focused Organizations:**

Elizabeth Glaser Pediatric AIDS Foundation: Works to eliminate pediatric AIDS and provides HIV care and treatment to mothers and children.

UNICEF: While broader in focus, UNICEF supports programs addressing pediatric HIV/AIDS globally.

- **Online Platforms and Initiatives:**

RED Campaign: Partners with various brands to raise funds for the Global Fund to fight AIDS, Tuberculosis, and Malaria.

Elton John AIDS Foundation: Established by the iconic musician, this foundation supports innovative HIV prevention and service programs.

Ways to contribute:

Regular Donations: Committing to regular donations, even small ones, can have a cumulative and sustained impact.

Employer Matching Programs: Check if your employer offers donation matching programs, which can effectively double your contribution.

Legacy Giving: Including charitable donations in your will or estate planning allows for a lasting impact.

In-kind donations: Donating goods or services can be valuable. For instance, supporting a local clinic with medical supplies or offering free services for a fundraising event

Social Media Advocacy: Amplify the impact of your contribution by leveraging social media to raise awareness and encourage others to join the cause.

Before contributing, it's important to research and ensure that the organization or initiative aligns with your values, operates transparently, and has a positive track record. Whether through fundraising events, regular donations, or volunteering time and skills, everyone can play a role in supporting the ongoing efforts to combat HIV/AIDS.

Advocacy and policy change

Advocacy and policy change are critical components in the ongoing efforts to combat HIV/AIDS. Effective advocacy involves raising awareness, influencing public opinion, and engaging with policymakers to bring about changes in laws, regulations, and public health practices. Here's an overview of how advocacy and policy change contribute to the fight against HIV/AIDS:

Advocacy Initiatives:

- **Raising Awareness:**
Community Education: Advocacy begins with educating communities about HIV/AIDS, its transmission, treatment, and prevention. Awareness campaigns help reduce stigma and discrimination.

Media Engagement: Utilizing various media channels, including social media, to disseminate accurate information and share personal stories that humanize the impact of HIV/AIDS

- **Challenging Stigma and Discrimination:**

Anti-Stigma Campaigns: Advocacy efforts aim to challenge and eliminate stigmatizing beliefs and discriminatory practices associated with HIV/AIDS.

Legal Protections: Advocates work towards the implementation and enforcement of legal protections against discrimination based on HIV status.

- **Promoting Testing and Treatment:**

Access to Testing: Advocacy for widespread access to HIV testing, emphasizing the importance of knowing one's status for prevention and early treatment.

Treatment Access: Advocating for policies that ensure affordable and accessible antiretroviral therapy (ART) for all individuals living with HIV

- **Prevention Strategies:**

Condom Distribution Programs: Advocacy for the distribution of condoms as part of comprehensive HIV prevention strategies

Needle Exchange Programs: Advocating for harm reduction strategies, including needle exchange programs, to reduce the transmission of HIV among injection drug users

Policy Change Initiatives:

- **Legislative Advocacy:**

Anti-Discrimination Laws: Advocating for and supporting the implementation of laws that protect individuals living with HIV from discrimination in various aspects of life, including employment and healthcare.

Access to Healthcare: Lobbying for policies that ensure affordable and accessible healthcare services for all, including comprehensive HIV/AIDS care.

- **Budget Advocacy:**

Allocations for HIV/AIDS Programs: Advocating for government budget allocations to support HIV prevention, treatment, research, and community-based programs

International Aid Advocacy: Encouraging governments to allocate funds for international aid programs focused on global HIV/AIDS prevention and treatment efforts

- **Community Engagement:**

Community-Based Research: Advocacy for policies that support community-based research, ensuring that affected communities actively participate in and benefit from research initiatives.

Inclusion in Decision-Making: Advocacy for policies that involve individuals living with HIV in decision-making processes related to their care and wellbeing.

- **International Collaboration:**

Global Health Policy Advocacy: Engaging in international advocacy efforts to promote policies that support global health initiatives, including those focused on HIV/AIDS

Trade Agreements and Access to Medications: Advocacy for trade policies that prioritize access to affordable medications, including antiretroviral drugs

- **Criminal Justice Reform:**

Decriminalization of HIV: advocacy for the repeal of laws that criminalize HIV transmission or exposure, recognizing that criminalization can deter individuals from seeking testing and treatment.

Ways Individuals Can Engage in Advocacy:

Contacting elected officials:

Writing letters, making phone calls, or meeting with elected officials to express support for HIV/AIDS-related policies and funding

Participating in Advocacy Organizations:

Joining or supporting organizations that focus on HIV/AIDS advocacy allows individuals to contribute to collective efforts.

Educating the Public:

Using personal experiences, knowledge, and platforms to educate the public about HIV/AIDS and advocate for evidence-based policies

Participating in Public Hearings and Consultations:

Attending public hearings and consultations on relevant policies to voice concerns, provide input, and advocate for specific measures

Collaborating with NGOs and Community Groups:

Partnering with nongovernmental organizations (NGOs) and community groups involved in HIV/AIDS advocacy to amplify impact

Advocacy and policy change are ongoing processes that require sustained efforts from individuals, communities, and organizations. By engaging in advocacy, individuals contribute to creating an environment that supports comprehensive HIV prevention, treatment, and care, which helps reduce the impact of the epidemic on affected populations.

CHAPTER 13: RESOURCES AND APPENDICES

Glossary of HIV-Related Terms:

1. **HIV (Human Immunodeficiency Virus)**: The virus that attacks the immune system, specifically CD4 cells (T cells), and can lead to AIDS.

2. **AIDS (Acquired Immunodeficiency Syndrome)**: The advanced stage of HIV infection, characterized by a severe depletion of the immune system and the occurrence of opportunistic infections or cancers.

3. **Antiretroviral Therapy (ART)**: A combination of medications used to slow down the progression of HIV and improve the health of individuals living with the virus.

4. **CD4 Cell Count**: A measure of the number of CD4 cells in a sample of blood, which indicates the health of the immune system.

5. **Viral load**: The amount of HIV in the blood, measured to assess the effectiveness of antiretroviral therapy.

6. **Pre-Exposure Prophylaxis (PrEP): medications** taken by HIVnegative individuals to prevent HIV infection

7. **Post-exposure Prophylaxis (PEP)**: Emergency medication taken after potential exposure to HIV to prevent infection.

8. **Seroconversion**: The period during which a person's blood changes from HIV-negative to HIV positive, usually accompanied by flu like symptoms.

9. **Undetectable Viral Load**: The level of HIV in the blood is so low that it cannot be detected by standard tests. Individuals with an undetectable viral load are less likely to transmit the virus.

10. **Opportunistic Infections**: Infections that take advantage of a weakened immune system, common in individuals with advanced HIV/AIDS.

List of Organizations and Hotlines:

1. amfAR (The Foundation for AIDS Research):

Website:

https://www.amfar.org/

2. UNAIDS (Joint United Nations Programme on HIV/AIDS):

Website:

https://www.unaids.org/

3. GMHC (Gay Men's Health Crisis):

Website:

https://www.gmhc.org/

4. AVAC (Global Advocacy for HIV Prevention):

Website:

https://www.avac.org/

5. Elizabeth Glaser Pediatric AIDS Foundation:

Website:

https://www.pedaids.org/

6. UNICEF (United Nations International Children's Emergency Fund):

Website:

https://www.unicef.org/

7. Treatment Action Group (TAG):
  Website:
https://www.treatmentactiongroup.org/

8. RED Campaign:
  Website: https://www.red.org/

9. Elton John AIDS Foundation:
  Website:
https://www.eltonjohnaidsfoundation.org/

10. National AIDS Hotline (USA):
  Hotline: 1800CDCINFO (18002324636)

11. The Trevor Project (LGBTQ+ Support):
  Hotline: 18664887386

Recommended Books, Websites, and Documentaries:

Books:

1. "And the Band Played On" by Randy Shilts:

A Comprehensive History of the Early Years of the AIDS Epidemic

2. "The Wisdom of Whores" by Elizabeth Pisani:

Explores the global response to the AIDS epidemic from a public health perspective.

3. "The AIDS Conspiracy: Science Fights Back" by Nicoli Nattrass:

Examines the origins of AIDS denialism and its impact on public health.

Websites:

1. HIV.gov:

https://www.hiv.gov/

A comprehensive resource for HIV information, prevention, testing, treatment, and support

2. TheBody:

https://www.thebody.com/

Provides information on HIV/AIDS, treatment options, and living with the virus.

Documentaries:

1. "How to Survive a Plague" (2012):

Chronicles the efforts of activists in the early years of the AIDS epidemic to advocate for better treatment options.

2. "United in Anger: A History of ACT UP" (2012):

Explores the history of the AIDS Coalition to Unleash Power (ACT UP) and its impact on HIV/AIDS activism.

3. "The Normal Heart" (2014):

Based on Larry Kramer's play, it provides a fictionalized account of the early years of the AIDS epidemic in New York City.

These resources offer a mix of educational content, personal narratives, and historical perspectives on HIV/AIDS. They can be valuable for individuals seeking a deeper understanding of the epidemic and its impact on individuals and communities.

CHAPTER 14: CONCLUSION AND CALL TO ACTION

Conclusion:

In conclusion, HIV/AIDS remains a global health challenge that demands ongoing attention, commitment, and collective action. The journey from the early days of the epidemic to the present has seen remarkable strides in understanding, prevention, and treatment. However, the persistence of new infections, lingering stigma, and the need for universal access to care underscore the importance of sustained efforts.

The Importance of HIV Prevention and Awareness:

Public Health Imperative: HIV prevention is not just a matter of personal health but a public health imperative. By preventing new infections, we contribute to healthier communities and a stronger global society.

Stigma Reduction: Increased awareness and education play a crucial role in reducing stigma and discrimination associated with HIV/AIDS. Creating an environment of understanding and empathy is essential for supporting individuals living with the virus.

Treatment Access: Prevention efforts go hand in hand with ensuring universal access to effective treatment. Early detection, coupled with timely and affordable antiretroviral therapy, not only saves lives but also reduces the risk of transmission.

Global Solidarity: The fight against HIV/AIDS is a global endeavor that requires solidarity. By working together across borders, we can share knowledge, resources, and best practices to address the diverse challenges posed by the epidemic.

Call to Action:

Get Educated: Knowledge is a powerful tool in the fight against HIV/AIDS. Stay informed about the latest developments in prevention, treatment, and research. Share this knowledge with others to contribute to a well-informed and empowered community.

Promote Testing and Early Detection: Encourage regular HIV testing for yourself and others. Early detection allows for timely intervention, reducing the impact of the virus on health and preventing further transmission.

Support HIV/AIDS Organizations: Contribute your time, skills, or financial resources to organizations dedicated to HIV/AIDS prevention, treatment, and support. Your support can make a tangible difference in the lives of individuals and communities affected by the virus.

Advocate for Policy Change: Engage with policymakers to advocate for policies that promote HIV prevention, treatment access, and the protection of the rights of individuals living with HIV. Your voice can be a catalyst for positive change.

Combat Stigma: Actively challenge and combat stigma and discrimination associated with HIV/AIDS. Foster a culture of inclusivity, understanding, and support within your community.

Engage in Safe Practices: Practice and promote safer sex practices, use of condoms, and other preventive measures.

By taking responsibility for your own health, you contribute to the broader effort of preventing new infections.

Stay Informed about Research: Stay abreast of ongoing research and breakthroughs in HIV/AIDS. Support and advocate for scientific endeavors that contribute to better prevention methods, treatment options, and, ultimately, finding a cure.

Closing Thoughts:

As we reflect on the progress made in the fight against HIV/AIDS, it's essential to recognize that the journey is far from over. Every individual has a role to play in creating a world free from the burdens of this epidemic. By staying informed, advocating for change, and supporting one another, we can collectively work towards the goal of ending HIV/AIDS, ensuring a healthier, more compassionate world for generations to come. The time to act is now. Get involved, make a difference, and be a part of the movement to end HIV/AIDS.